José A. Tapia
Chernobyl and the Mortality Crisis in Eastern Europe and the Former USSR

De Gruyter Contemporary Social Sciences

—

Volume 11

José A. Tapia

Chernobyl and the Mortality Crisis in Eastern Europe and the Former USSR

—

DE GRUYTER

ISBN 978-3-11-153072-7
e-ISBN (PDF) 978-3-11-076178-8
e-ISBN (EPUB) 978-3-11-076189-4
ISSN 2747-5689
e-ISSN 2747-5697

Library of Congress Control Number: 2022939905

Bibliographic information published by the Deutsche Nationalbibliothek
The Deutsche Nationalbibliothek lists this publication in the Deutsche
Nationalbibliografie; detailed bibliographic data are available on the internet at http://
dnb.dnb.de.

www.degruyter.com

Acknowledgements

I am grateful to several persons who gave me very valuable insights and comments on the drafts that led up to this book. Fernando J. García López from the National Epidemiology Center of the Instituto de Salud Carlos III in Madrid encouraged me to pursue this project, read in a short notice the whole manuscript of the book and convinced me I had to explain better or more in detail quite a number of issues. Kate Brown, Amy Auchincloss, Tomás Ortín, and Keith Meyers were very helpful in giving me key references or critical insights on different aspects of the book. Edward Ionides, my coauthor for many years, gave me in his typical terse style highly valuable comments on earlier manuscripts that helped me focus the whole project. Isabella Diez Imbriaco helped a lot with the references. Last but not least, Ana Diez Roux read the manuscripts that led to the final product and gave me a lot of useful comments—not to mention her support in so many other aspects of my life. My thanks to all of them. Of course, the usual disclaimer applies, and I am the only one responsible for any inconvenient, impolite, or incorrect assertions and views that I know may be present in this book.

https://doi.org/10.1515/9783110761788-001

About the author

José A. Tapia Granados is a professor of politics at Drexel University, Philadelphia. With degrees in medicine, public health, and economics, he worked formerly for the Spanish Social Security system, the publishing industry, the World Health Organization, and the University of Michigan. He coauthored with Rolando Astarita *La Gran Depresión y el capitalismo del siglo XXI* (Madrid, Catarata, 2011) and is the author of *Rentabilidad, inversión y crisis* (Madrid, Maia, 2017) and *Cambio climático: ¿Qué hacer?* (Madrid, Maia, 2021). His papers have appeared in *PNAS, International Journal of Epidemiology, Lancet, Environmental Science & Policy, Journal of Health Economics, Social Science and Medicine, Demography, American Journal of Epidemiology, International Journal of Public Health,* and other journals. He presently teaches courses on political economy of climate change, international political economy, political parties, and social development. He has written on music and on political and social issues in *MundoClásico, Mientras Tanto, The Brooklyn Rail, Capitalism-Nature-Socialism*, and other venues.

https://doi.org/10.1515/9783110761788-002

Preface

The idea to write this essay came to me about one year before the COVID-19 pandemic, when I read the books on Chernobyl by Svetlana Alexievich and Kate Brown. I had been convinced since long ago that the mortality crisis that occurred in Eastern Europe and the republics of the old Soviet Union in the last decade of the 20th century is one of the most important health disasters of the modern era. After reading the books by Alexievich and Brown it occurred to me that Chernobyl could be very well one of the factors explaining the extreme severity and the protracted duration of that health crisis in which mortality rates skyrocketed in the countries of Eastern Europe and the republics that had been part of the USSR. I did some preliminary research looking at mortality rates and birth rates and what I found convinced me that the hypothesis was worth investigating. I presented my research at a seminar at the National Epidemiology Center of the Instituto de Salud Carlos III, in Madrid, in February 2020, immediately before the COVID-19 pandemic hit us all in the face. In that seminar I noted many things that need to be developed and refined. In the months following the seminar I tried to synthesize my thoughts in a manuscript that could become a journal paper, but there were many things to say, and the project grew into a book project that, right in the middle of the COVID-19 pandemic, Walter de Gruyter GmbH evaluated and agreed to publish.

After reading a draft of this book, Edward Ionides said to me in an email that people should read my Chernobyl hypothesis from the perspective that some unknown fraction of the demographic crisis affecting death rates could plausibly be due to radioactivity. From this "natural experiment" with so many other things changing at the same time, it is not possible to make a strong argument based only on the data presented here that the only plausible cause of the mortality crisis that started in these countries in the late 1980s is Chernobyl. But the value of the book is, Ionides said, "to put the different strands of the argument (including some that are not so well known) together, to support a hypothesis but not to claim that the hypothesis is fully proved or disproved by the evidence. In the unhappy event that the world gets more such experiments, it will be useful to bear in mind this possibility." I believe these remarks are a very good introduction to this book.

My basic claim is that the 1986 Chernobyl disaster is likely a significant causal component of the mortality upturn that started in the countries of Eastern Europe, the Balkans, and the Soviet Union in the late 1980s, grew to a full mortality crisis in the 1990s, and in some countries extended beyond 2000. All these countries were at the time going through a difficult period of social, political, and eco-

https://doi.org/10.1515/9783110761788-003

nomic unrest. Using a variety of approaches, I try to show the plausibility of the hypothesis that the mortality effects of the radiation released by the Chernobyl disaster are a non-negligible component of this mortality crisis. I use demographic indicators (life expectancy at birth, birth rates and sex ratios at birth) to show the major changes in the population dynamics of the countries of the old Soviet bloc that occurred at the time of Chernobyl or soon after. It seems to me the information I present here is highly suggestive of the fact that the radioactive rainfall caused by the Chernobyl disaster had a discernible influence in the evolution of demographic rates in the countries of the old Soviet bloc, particularly in Belarus, Ukraine, Russia, the Baltic republics and Bulgaria. However, because the information at hand is fragmentary and dispersed, and because the issue is very complex and requires examining many different factors, I have not attempted to make an estimate of the proportion of the excess mortality suffered by the countries of the old Soviet bloc since 1986 that can be attributed to the Chernobyl disaster. But I argue in the book that the contribution of that disaster to the mortality crisis in each country is very likely nontrivial. Whether that contribution amounts to 2%, 11% or some other number, it is a task for future research.

I have tried to address an audience of people with diverse backgrounds who will be interested in the issue stated in the title of the book. Researchers in public health, epidemiologists and demographers are the ones who will best understand my reasoning, but I have tried to explain each specialized concept that I use so that the text is understandable by an audience that is not specialized and may have just a minimal background in natural science or social science. I have tried to be as clear as possible in explaining technical issues related to radiation and radioactivity, but I assume the reader has a basic knowledge of science, particularly about physics (so that he knows for instance that radioisotopes and radionuclides are the same thing) and biology (so that she knows for example that mutations of the genetic material are just alterations of the DNA).

In this book the spelling Chernobyl, more common in English and based on Latin transliteration of the Cyrillic Russian spelling, is used rather than Chornobyl, based on Ukrainian spelling. Since this preface is being written at the time the Russian army is invading Ukraine—indeed the Chernobyl area in north Ukraine is now occupied by Russian troops—perhaps it is proper to mention that, of course, this choice of words merely reflects the most well-known term in the English-speaking world and does not imply any preference for Russian spelling.

The radionuclide cesium-137, also spelled caesium-137, is one of the most important components of the radioactive fallout from the Chernobyl disaster. The two spellings are almost equally frequent in the scientific literature that I have used and I have not tried to avoid the use of both spellings in this book.

Contents

Abbreviations

The following list of abbreviations includes all the acronyms and abbreviations used in the text. Many of them like USSR, US, WHO, PR, ENT, CV, IQ, km, or CVD refer to states, countries, agencies of the United Nations (UN) system, or common concepts of everyday life or the scientific language, they are relatively well known for anyone who reads in English and will be used without explanation in the text. They are explained here considering that many readers of this book may not be as familiar with English. The list also includes abbreviations that will be used in the text but will be explained when they appear for the first time. For the definition of units such as curie or sievert, see Appendix A.

°C	degrees centigrade (Celsius)
BEAR	biological effects of atomic radiation
BEIR	biological effects of ionizing radiation
BMJ	British Medical Journal
Bq	becquerel
Ci	curie
CLL	chronic lymphocytic leukemia
CPSU	Communist Party of the Soviet Union
CV	curriculum vitae
CVD	cardiovascular disease
DNA	deoxyribonucleic acid
DREF	dose-rate effectiveness factor,
DDREF	dose and dose-rate effectiveness factor
ENT	ear, nose, and throat
ERR	excess relative risk
e.g.	*exempli gratia* in Latin, meaning "for example."
FAO	UN Food and Agriculture Organization
Gy	gray
FDA	Food and Drug Administration (US government agency)
IAEA	International Atomic Energy Agency
ICRP	International Commission on Radiological Protection
i.e.	*id est*, Latin for "that is"
IQ	intelligence quotient
JAMA	Journal of the American Medical Association
km	kilometer
LEB	life expectancy at birth
LET	linear energy transfer
LNT model	linear no threshold model
MBq	megabecquerel
mGy	milligray
mSv	millisievert
NIH	National Institutes of Health (US government agency)
OCHA	UN Office for the Coordination of Humanitarian Affairs
PI	principal investigator
PNAS	Proceedings of the National Academy of Sciences of the USA

https://doi.org/10.1515/9783110761788-004

PR	public relations
Sv	sievert
UNDP	UN Development Programme
UNSCEAR	UN Scientific Committee on the Effects of Atomic Radiation
WHO	World Health Organization
US	United States of America
USSR	Union of Soviet Socialist Republics (Soviet Union)

Chapter 1
Introduction

The breakdown of the Soviet bloc including the collapse of the USSR itself and the disappearance of the centrally planned economies in Eastern Europe and the Balkans was the most important historical event at the end of the 20th century. This is a generally agreed upon and known fact. Much less known is the fact that the mortality crisis that occurred in the countries involved in the transition to a market economy was arguably the major peacetime health crisis of recent decades.[1]

Life expectancy at birth (LEB), that is, expectation of life at age 0, e_0 in demographic notation, is often used as a major indicator of population health. LEB at a given year is fully determined by the mortality rates registered that year, as it is the average length of life of a hypothetical cohort exposed from birth to the death of all its members to the age-specific mortality rates observed that year.[2] Worldwide, during the 20th century, mortality rates showed a declining long term trend and consequently, LEB increased in almost every country (Fig. 1.1). This general trend was only interrupted by periods of war, genocide, major political repression, or famine.[3] For instance, LEB dropped in 1918 in virtually all countries of the world because of the world flu pandemic, misnamed "the Spanish flu": between 1917 and 1918, in Sweden LEB dropped by 9.1 years (from 58.8 to 49.7), while in Switzerland it dropped 9.5 years (from 55.8 to 46.3), in Iceland by 7.9 years (59.0 to 51.1), in the Netherlands by 8.0 years (55.6 to 47.6) and in Spain by 12.2 years (42.6 to 30.4). During the 20th century male LEB also showed major declines in times of war. Thus, for example, between 1922 and 2016, LEB for British males grew from 55.2 to 79.2 years, but during World War II it declined from 61.4 years in 1939 to 58.0 years in 1941 and the prewar level was not reat-

---

1 The burden of premature mortality caused by this crisis can be estimated in several million deaths, as the crisis extended into the 21st century and it was estimated that only in the period 1989–1996 in Eastern Europe and the countries of the old USSR 3 million premature deaths had occurred. At the time of this writing, it is estimated that worldwide the COVID-19 pandemic has caused at least 6 million premature deaths.
2 This is what demographers call period LEB. Cohort LEB is the mean length of life of all individuals born in a given year, and obviously can be calculated only for years very long in the past.
3 Mackenbach (2013), "Political conditions and life expectancy in Europe, 1900–2008", *Social Science & Medicine* 82, 134–146; Tapia Granados (2013), "Repression, famines, and wars: Major impacts of politics on population health", *Social Science & Medicine* 86, 103–106.

https://doi.org/10.1515/9783110761788-005

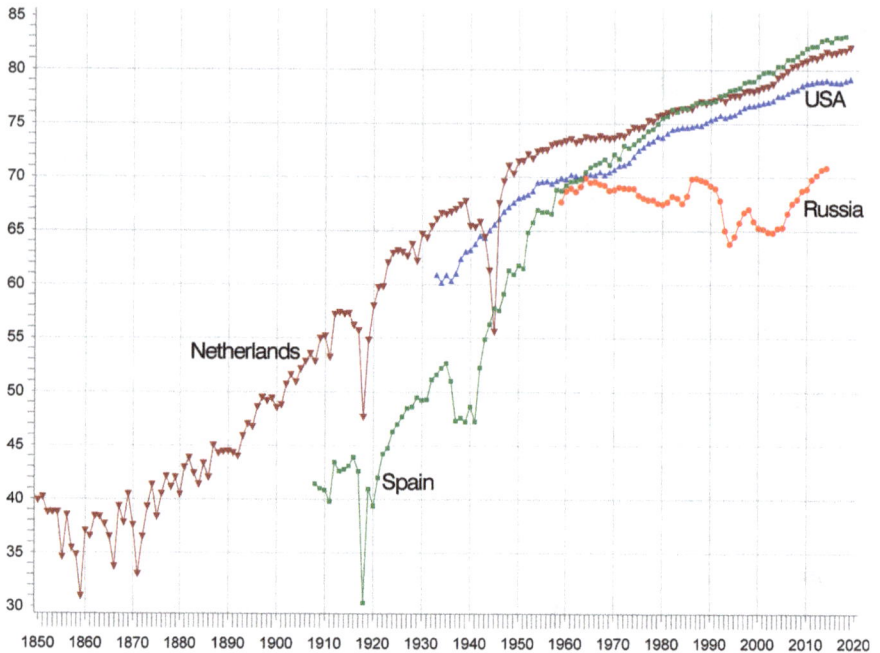

Fig. 1.1: Life expectancy at birth (LEB, in years) in four countries for which reliable data exist for specific periods. Note the major drops in LEB caused by the world flu pandemic in 1918, the Spanish civil war starting in 1936, and the German occupation of the Netherlands in 1940–1945, during World War II. Russia is a very special case concerning the evolution of LEB since the mid-1960s. Author's elaboration from data in the Human Mortality Database.

tained until 1945.[4] According to the estimates of Russian demographers published after the breakdown of the USSR, in the European part of the Soviet Union, LEB for males declined from 36.5 years in 1928 to 31.1 in 1932 and to a stunning 10.3 years in 1933.[5] This happened in the context of major political repression and compulsory collectivization of agriculture which evolved into a major famine in Western areas of the USSR. Genocides like those occurring in Cambodia in the 1970s and in Ruanda in the 1990s, and famines like those of 1942 in Bengal under British colonial rule or in the Netherlands in 1944–1945

---

4 The LEB figures cited or used for graphs in this chapter are from the Human Mortality Database (University of California at Berkeley, Max Planck Institute for Demographic Research), except when other source is indicated.

5 Haynes & Husan (2003), *A century of state murder? Death and policy in 20th-century Russia*.

under Nazi occupation where also associated with significant declines in LEB.[6] Thus in the Netherlands, LEB dropped from 67.7 years in 1939 to 65.4 years in 1940, when the German occupation started (Fig.1.1). It declined even further to 61.3 years in 1944, and then to 55.6 years in 1945, when the country suffered a major winter famine; with the end of the German occupation and the war LEB recovered quickly, gaining 11.9 years between 1945 and 1946, to reach 67.5 years in 1946.

The decades following World War II saw generalized and steadily declining mortality rates and increasing levels of LEB all over the world. However, from the mid-1960s, the countries of Western Europe, North America, and other high-income nations saw a continuation of improving mortality conditions, while in East and Central Europe, male mortality began to deteriorate and LEB stagnated or even declined (Fig. 1.1).[7] In Central Europe for example, since the mid-1960s a major divergence appeared in the evolution of LEB in the centrally planned economies belonging at the time to the Soviet bloc or to the Federal Yugoslavia, and the countries with a market economy, so that in 1980 a wide gap had opened between Switzerland's and Austria's LEB and that of the neighboring Chechia and Slovakia (at the time united in Czechoslovakia), and Hungary (Fig. 1.2). Illustrative of the same phenomenon is the fact that in

the early 1960s Russia, the US, and Spain had similar levels of LEB, while in 1980 Russia's LEB was 9 years below the LEB of Spain and 8 years below the LEB of the US (Fig. 1.1). Overall, since the mid-1960s there was a remarkable stagnation and even decline in LEB in the republics of Eastern Europe and the USSR.[8] Though this negative evolution somewhat weakened in the early 1980s, when there were gains in LEB in many of these countries, the evolution of LEB deteriorated again at the end of the 1980s and in the early 1990s, in the early transition to a market economy. As Andrea Cornia put it in 2000, the tendency of mortality rates to increase intensified sharply from 1989 so that despite widespread popular expectations "for substantial improvements in living standards and health conditions, the transition to the market economy" was "accompanied by a sharp demographic crisis which [...] featured *inter alia* very large and sud-

---

6 According to data reported by the World Bank which are known to be quite rough approximations, Ruanda's LEB that had been 51.7 years in 1985 dropped steadily in the following years to reach a minimum of 26.2 years in 1993; only in 2003 LEB recovered over pre-genocide levels (data.worldbank.org/indicator/SP.DYN.LE00.IN). From the same source, Cambodia's LEB was 42.6 years in 1968; then steadily decreased in the years of war and genocide to a minimum of 18.9 in 1977.

7 Tomka (2013), *A social history of 20th-century Europe*, 29 – 30.

8 Cockerham (1999), *Health and social change in Russia and Eastern Europe*.

den rises in mortality rates." Because of the extent, suddenness and causes of death, the mortality crisis of Eastern Europe after 1989 was without precedent in the European peacetime history of the 20th century.[9]

The countries affected and the characteristics of the mortality crisis

The mortality crisis, involving significant drops in LEB, took place in the republics of the Soviet Union (Figures 1.1, 1.2 and 1.3), as well as in the countries of the Soviet bloc (Fig. 1.4) and the Balkans (Fig. 1.5) coinciding or following the remov-

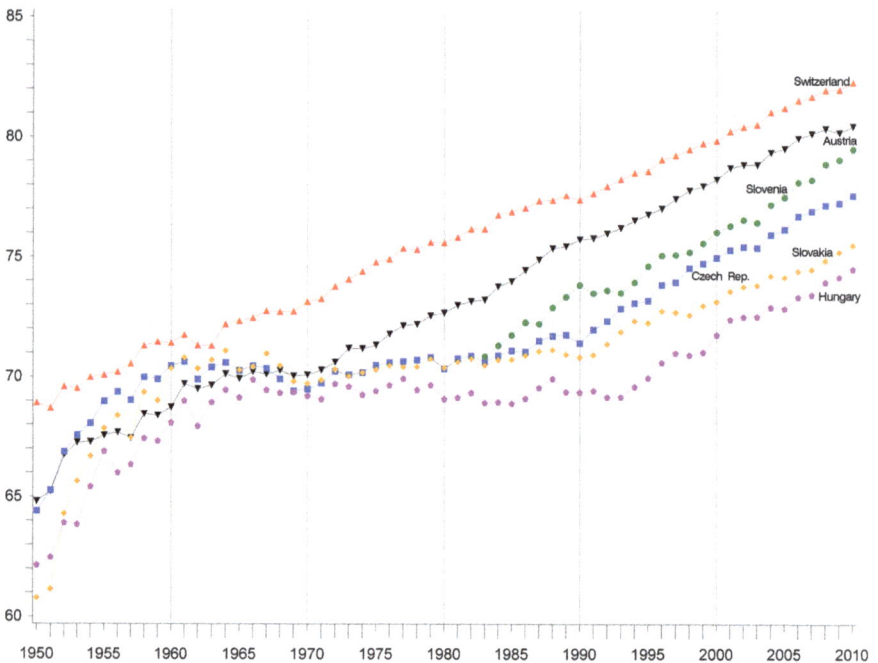

Fig. 1.2: Life expectancy at birth in six countries of Central Europe. Note that until 1990 the Czech Republic and Slovakia were part of Czechoslovakia, while Slovenia was part of Yugoslavia. Author's elaboration from data in the HFA database, WHO-Europe.

---

9 Cornia & Paniccià (2000), *The mortality crisis in transitional economies.*

al of communist parties from government (around 1990) and the transition of the planned economies into a market system.[10] The countries that suffered this mortality crisis were those that had been parts of the USSR, allies of the Soviet Union in the so-called Soviet bloc — which militarily corresponded to the Warsaw Pact —, republics of the Federation of Yugoslavia, and isolated countries like Albania — for a time the European follower of the Chinese variety of Marxism-Leninism.

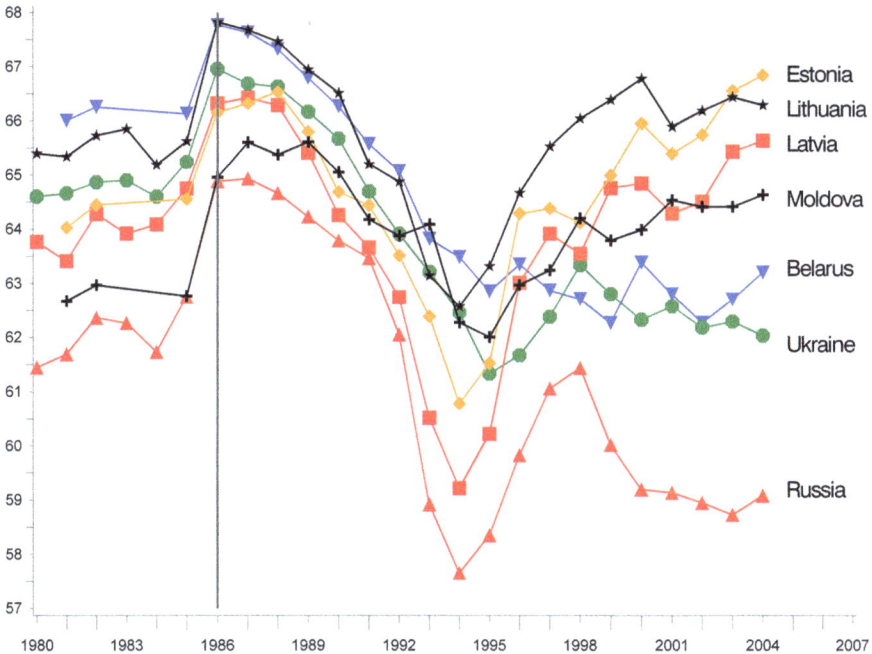

Fig. 1.3: Life expectancy at birth for males in the Western republics of the former USSR, 1980–2004. The vertical line marks 1986, the year in which the Chernobyl disaster occurred. Author's elaboration from data in the HFA database, WHO-Europe.

Mortality, particularly of men, had evolved poorly in most countries of the Soviet bloc since the 1970s.[11] For instance, as estimated by Stephen Kunitz in 1994, the

---

10 Cornia & Paniccià (2000), *The mortality crisis;* Stillman (2006), "Health and nutrition in Eastern Europe and the former Soviet Union during the decade of transition," *Economics & Human Biology* 4(1), 104–146.
11 Cockerham (1999), *Health and social change.*

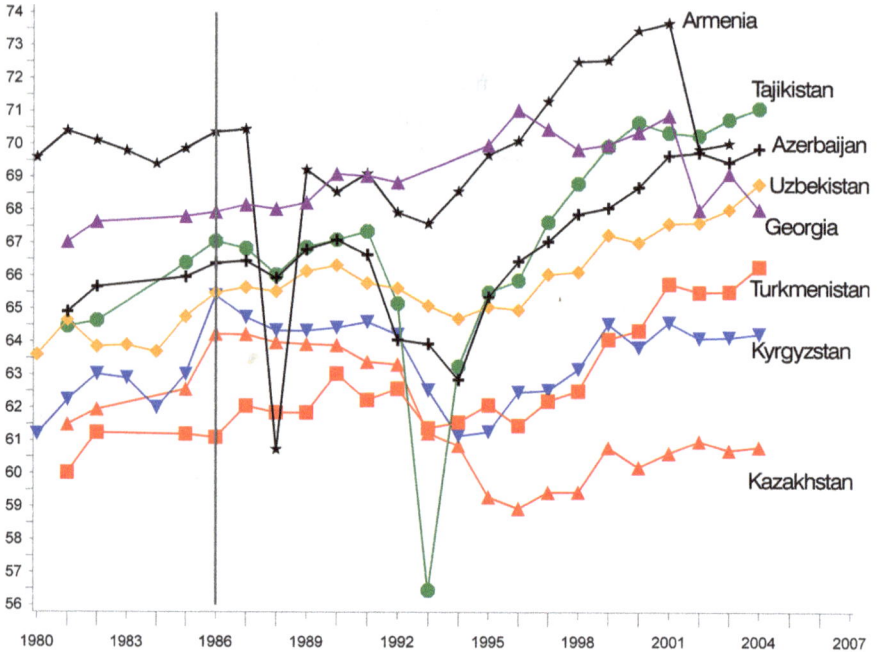

Fig. 1.4: Life expectancy at birth (LEB, years) for males in the republics of the former USSR in the Caucasus or Central Asia, 1980–2004. The vertical line marks 1986, the year in which the Chernobyl disaster occurred. The drop of LEB in Armenia in 1988 was caused by an earthquake that killed thousands of people, most children. Author's elaboration from data in the HFA database, WHO-Europe.

USSR male LEB that had gained annually 0.3 years in the period between the mid-1950s and the mid-1970s, gained annually only 0.11 years in the period from the mid-1970s to the mid-1980s. In these two periods, the annual gains in US male LEB had been respectively 0.20 and 0.33 years, while in Western Europe they had been respectively 0.28 and 0.47 years, and in Southern Europe they had been 0.64 and 0.35 years.[12] But the evolution of mortality in the countries of the Soviet bloc worsened considerably in the late 1980s and early 1990s (see Figs. 1.1 to 1.3). Indeed, the mortality crisis as defined for instance by Cornia and Paniccià roughly coincided with the quick transformation of these countries into market economies, a period of sudden and quite chaotic change, often described as "the

12 Kunitz (1994), "The value of particularism in the study of the cultural, social and behavioral determinants of mortality", Table 9.3.

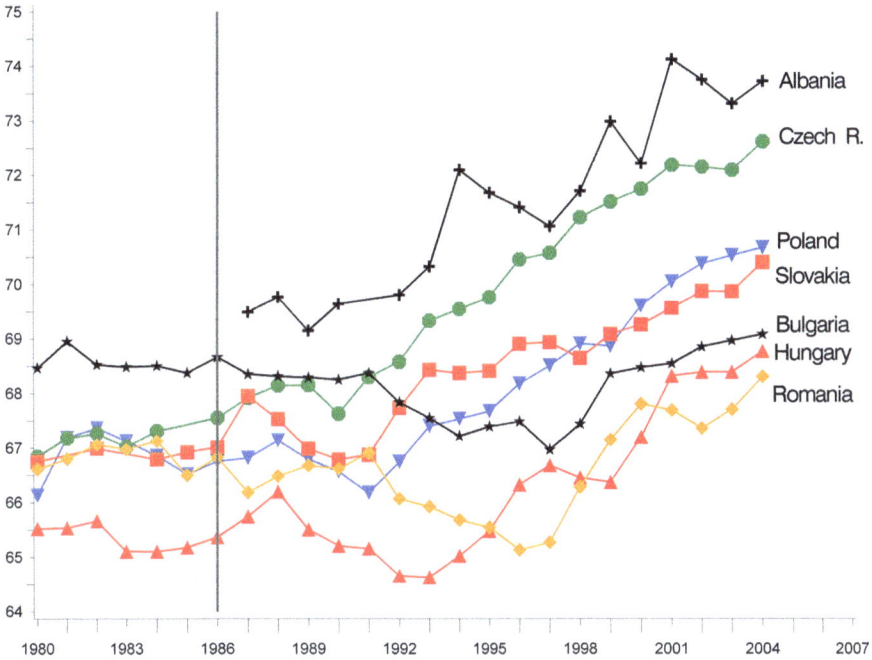

Fig. 1.5: Life expectancy at birth for males in the Eastern Europe nations of the Soviet bloc, plus Albania, 1980–2004. The vertical line marks 1986, the year in which the Chernobyl disaster occurred. Author's elaboration from data in the HFA database, WHO-Europe.

transition from communism to capitalism." In this period some nations of Eastern Europe, the Balkans and the old Soviet Union reinstated civil liberties long time suppressed by communist parties in government, while others — e.g., Belarus, Kazakhstan, Kyrgyzstan, Uzbekistan, and Turkmenistan — remained under autocratic regimes, and still others — e.g., Tajikistan, Armenia, Azerbaijan, Georgia, and the republics of the old Yugoslavia — entered periods of violent civil unrest and even war. The communist regime in East Germany collapsed in 1989, in December that year the demolition of the Berlin Wall started and in 1990 the German Democratic Republic ceased to exist by incorporation into the Federal Republic of Germany. LEB of East German men declined the year of the unification by 0.9 years (from 70.1 years in 1989 to 69.2 in 1992) and did not recover to the 1989 level until 1992 (when it reached 70.0 years). Before the unification, the East German male LEB had been increasing slowly, but the only period in

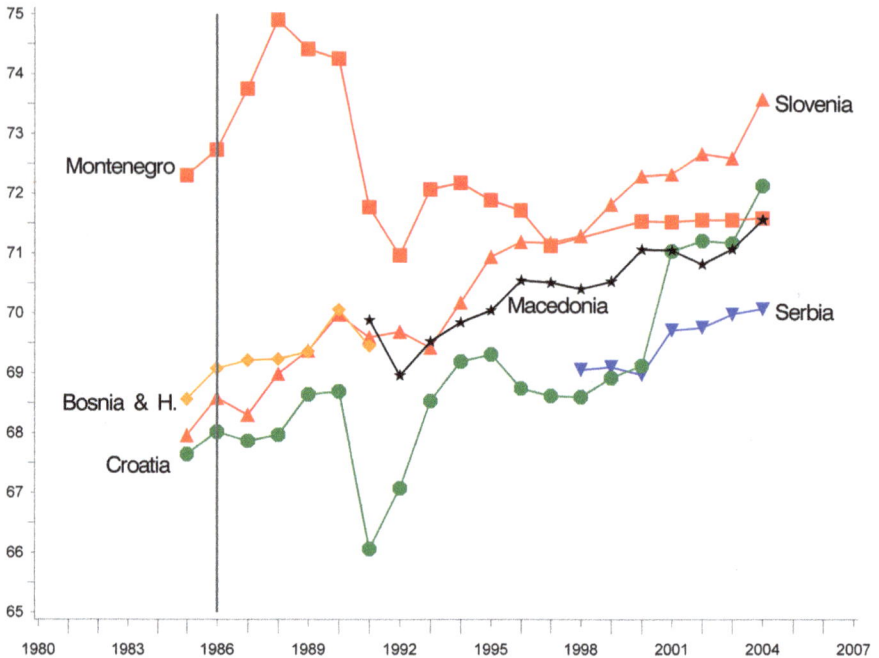

Fig. 1.6: Life expectancy at birth for males in the republics of the former Yugoslavia, 1980 – 2004. The vertical line marks 1986, the year in which the Chernobyl disaster occurred. Author's elaboration from data in the HFA database, WHO-Europe.

which it actually decreased, although it was a relatively small decrease, was after the collapse of the communist regime.[13]

At the time of the transition into a market economy in the early 1990s millions of people in the countries of the old Soviet bloc lost their jobs, their savings, their free health care, and often all of these. "Men in particular were unneeded by the state and by others around them. Work, for the first time in their lives, was no longer certain. In the context of hyperinflation, salary arrears, forced retirements, and layoffs in the early 1990s, men were unable to fulfill their role as breadwinners."[14] Though this was written on Russia, it would be applicable too to the other republics of the USSR and Eastern Europe. Furthermore, those whose national identity was linked to the countries of Yugoslavia, Czechoslovakia, or the Soviet Union, ceased having a nation in the 1990s and were

---

13 Cockerham (1999), *Health and social change*, 241.
14 Parsons (2014), *Dying unneeded: The cultural context of the Russian mortality crisis*, 172.

forced to adopt a different national identity.[15] These are powerful sources of social stress, that very likely had a major role in the mortality increase of these
years.

Tab. 1.1: Length and depth of the mortality crisis as measured by life expectancy for males
(LEBm) in the fifteen republics of the former USSR[a].

	A	B	C	D	E	F = E-A	G = B-D
	Peak		Trough				
Country	Year	LEBm	Year	LEBm	Recovery	Length	Depth
Georgia	1990	69.1	2002	68.0	1995	5	1.1
Tajikistan	1991	67.4	1993	56.4	1997	6	10.9
Azerbaijan	1990	67.1	1994	62.9	1998	8	4.2
Turkmenistan	1990	63.0	1993	61.4	1999	9	1.7
Uzbekistan	1990	66.3	1994	64.7	1999	9	1.6
Armenia	1987	70.5	1993	67.6	1997	10	2.9
Estonia	1988	66.5	1994	60.8	2004	16	5.8
Latvia	1987	66.4	1994	59.2	2008	21	7.2
Moldova	1989	65.6	1995	62.0	2011	22	3.6
Kyrgyzstan	1986	65.4	1994	61.1	2010	24	4.3
Kazakhstan	1986	64.2	1996	58.9	2011	25	5.3
Lithuania	1986	67.8	1994	62.6	2011	25	5.2
Russia	1987	64.9	1994	57.7	2013	26	7.3
Belarus	1986	67.8	1999	62.3	2014	28	5.5
Ukraine	1986	67.0	1995	61.3	2015	29	5.6

[a] The depth of the crisis is the difference between the highest (peak) value reached by LEBm
before the crisis and the lowest value (trough) reached by LEBm during the crisis. The length
of the crisis is the number of years between the year of the peak precrisis LEBm and the year
in which this LEBm was subsequently surpassed. Author's elaboration from data in the WHO-
HFA database. See Tab. C1 in Appendix C.

The mortality increases in this period were mostly due to rising rates of heart at-
tacks and other CVD, liver cirrhosis, suicide, homicide, and deaths due to injuries and poisoning, with male mortality much more affected than female mortality.[16] However, the depth and length of the mortality crisis varied considerably

---

15 This process was often extremely stressful — as superbly described for the case of the USSR
by the Nobel Prize winner Svetlana Alexievich in her book *Second-hand time*.
16 For that reason, the analysis here focuses on male LEB. In Appendix B, I show statistics for
female LEB and discuss some issues connected with the differential gender effect that the Chernobyl disaster may have had.

across countries (see Tab 1.1 and Tab 1.2). In East Germany, the Czech Republic, Slovakia, and Slovenia, the pre-transition levels of LEB that had been reached in 1987–1991 were regained in 1991–1994;[17] in Albania the pretransition peak in male LEB, 69.8 years, occurred in 1988 and in 1993 male LEB surpassed the pre-transition peak reaching 70.3 years, thus the crisis lasted 5 years; Croatia had a 4-year crisis (Tab. 1.2). But these quick recoveries appear to have been exceptions rather than the rule. Poland attained pre-transition levels of male LEB in 1993 and had had a peak in 1988, thus its crisis lasted 5 years; in Hungary the peak was in 1988 and the recovery in 1996, i.e., a crisis length of 8 years. Before the political transition, male LEB in Romania peaked at 66.7 in 1989 — the year in which the Ceaușescu were overthrown and executed — and surpassed this level in 1999, thus the crisis lasted 10 years; however, the length of the crisis is 16 years if we start counting in 1984 when male LEB had a local maximum at 67.1, that was only surpassed in 2000 when male LEB reached 67.8 years. In Bulgaria male LEB reached a maximum of 69.0 in 1981, level that was only surpassed in 2004; immediately before the transition to a market economy male LEB was 68.4 in 1991, a level that was surpassed at 68.5 in 2000; thus the mortality crisis lasted either 23 years or 9 years, depending how we count it. In the republics formerly part of Yugoslavia, information is too fragmentary to allow for proper comparisons, but the available data suggest a quite long mortality crisis.

The new independent republics formerly part of the USSR had generally much worse mortality crises (i.e., greater and longer declines in LEB) than the countries of Eastern Europe and the Balkans. Thus, in the three Baltic countries, pre-independence levels of male LEB were not surpassed until 2004 in Estonia, until 2008 in Latvia, and until 2011 in Lithuania, so that the mortality crises in these countries lasted 16, 21, and 25 years, respectively (Tab. 1.1). In most of the other republics of the former USSR it took several years, one decade or even two to recover the levels of male LEB that had been reached before the demise of the Soviet Union in 1991. Tajikistan recovered that level in 1997, Azerbaijan in 1998, Armenia in 1997, Turkmenistan in 1999, Kyrgyzstan in 2010, Moldova and Kazakhstan in 2011. The three ex-Soviet republics with the longest mortality crises were Russia, Belarus, and Ukraine, where the pre-independence levels of male LEB were reached respectively in 2013, 2014 and 2015. These data show the magnitude of the peacetime disaster of population health that in several of these countries extended well into the 21st century. Just for comparison it can be

---

17 Riphahn & Zimmermann (2000), "The mortality crisis in East Germany", in Cornia & Paniccià, eds, *The mortality crisis*, pp. 227–252; WHO Europe, European Health For All Database (HFA-DB). Cornia & Paniccià (2000), *The mortality crisis*.

Tab. 1.2: Length and depth of the mortality crisis as measured by life expectancy for males (LEBm) in the formerly planned economies of Eastern Europe and the Balkans[a].

	A	B	C	D	E	F = E-A	G=B-D
		Peak		Trough			
Country	Year	LEBm	Year	LEBm	Recovery	Length	Deepness
Czech Republic	1989	68.2	1990	67.6	1991	2	0.6
Albania	1988	69.8	1989	69.2	1993	5	0.6
Poland	1988	67.1	1991	66.1	1994	6	0.9
Croatia	1990	68.7	1991	66.1	1994	4	2.6
North Macedonia	1991	69.9	1992	69.0	1995	4	0.9
Slovenia	1990	70.0	1993	69.4	1994	4	0.6
Slovakia	1987	68.0	1992	66.8	1993	6	1.2
Hungary	1988	66.2	1993	64.6	1996	8	1.6
Romania	1984	67.1	1996	65.1	2000	16	2.0
Bulgaria	1981	69.0	1997	67.0	2004	23	2.0

[a] Length and depth of the crisis computed as in Tab. 1.1. Author's elaboration from data in the WHO-HFA database where data for Montenegro, Serbia, and Bosnia-Herzegovina are very incomplete so they are not included in this table. See also Tab. C2 in Appendix C.

cited that in Spain the peak LEB for males before the 1936–1939 civil war was 50.7 years, that correspond to the mortality rates of 1935, while the lowest male LEB caused by the killings in the war front and in the rearguard, 42.9 years, was registered in 1937, and the recovery to prewar levels occurred in 1943.[18] Thus the male mortality crisis caused by the Spanish civil war of 1936–1939 lasted 8 years and had a depth of 7.8 years, figures which look small compared with the Russian male mortality crisis of the transition that with an identical depth of 7.8 lasted however 26 years.

It can be argued that the 1990s political and economic transition in these countries was not always a peaceful or democratic one. Communist parties were removed from power relatively peacefully but in some countries like Romania government repression implied considerable violence. In some cases, the political systems that emerged were democratic regimes with civil liberties and governments elected peacefully in more or less free elections. But in other cases, for instance in several republics of the former Yugoslavia, as well as some countries of the Caucasus and Central Asia, war raged for years. With few exceptions, in

---

18 Data from the Human Mortality Database. See also Fig. 1.1 but note that the LEB figures there are for both males and females, not only males.

the ex-Soviet republics of Central Asia and the Western USSR, dictatorships with only a thin appearance of democracy were installed following the displacement of communist parties from power. In Russia a constitutional crisis in 1993 ended when troops loyal to President Yeltsin stormed the parliament building, after the parliament had impeached Yeltsin. Whatever the political regime after the political transition, as a rule all these countries quite quickly became market economies and, in the process, big opportunities for making money emerged and were taken advantage of by investors and businessmen. In a generalized process of privatization, former *apparatchiks*, that is, top level officers of the Communist Party often evolved to be the new oligarchs by becoming owners of economic resources formerly under state ownership and control.[19]

With low wages, very low or inexistent capital taxes, and scarce regulations for environmental or occupational health, in the 1990s Eastern Europe became the cradle where big fortunes and economic empires were born while the mortality crisis raged. It was estimated that in the period 1989–1996 the mortality crisis in Eastern Europe and the countries of the old USSR caused over 3 million extra deaths.[20] Only in Russia, it was estimated the mortality burden of the crisis in 1990–1998 was 3.4 million premature deaths.[21] Since the mortality crisis extended in many countries to the first and even to the second decade of the present century, these estimates are clearly just lower bounds.

Explanations of the mortality crisis

Despite the steady growth of the subdiscipline called social epidemiology, Western epidemiologists did not appear to have been particularly interested in studying the mortality crisis in transitional economies, as the years of increasing mortality in the old Soviet bloc were first called. This mortality crisis of the transition from Soviet communism to capitalism generated much less interest and publications than, for instance the differential frequency of morbidity or mortality in groups of the population of Western countries stratified by social class, ethnicity, employment conditions, or other social variables. Major works of hundreds of

---

19 Wedel (2001), *Collision and collusion: The strange case of western aid to Eastern Europe.*
20 Cornia & Paniccià (2000), *The mortality crisis*, vii.
21 Rosefield (2001), "Premature deaths: Russia's radical economic transition in Soviet perspective," *Europe-Asia Studies* 53(8), 1159–1176.

pages on social epidemiology did not mention the mortality crisis in the transitional economies of Eastern Europe or mention it just in passing.[22]

Demographers, medical sociologists, and economists were apparently more interested than epidemiologists in the mortality crisis of Eastern Europe. With the collaboration of health researchers and demographers from Bulgaria, the Czech Republic, Hungary, Poland, Romania, and Russia, the medical sociologist William Cockerham produced in 1999 the volume *Health and social change in Russia and Eastern Europe*, which opened by stating unambiguously that the decline in life expectancy in the former Soviet Union and Eastern Europe was "one of the most significant developments in world health in the late twentieth century". Cockerham explained how both presentations and private conversations in a meeting of the European Society of Health and Medical Sociology in Vienna in 1992 revealed to him that it was well known that levels of health and life expectancy were seriously declining in the former Soviet bloc, but "no one — from either the East or the West — could explain why this situation was occurring." That a group of industrialized countries under common circumstances suffered such a severe deterioration in public health was not only a health disaster for the peoples involved, but also an intriguing puzzle to be solved. The purpose of his book, said Cockerham, was to solve that puzzle.[23]

After a careful review of the evidence, Cockerham's conclusion was that unhealthy lifestyles were the primary social determinant of the higher death rates observed. However, following the views on *habitus* of the French sociologist Pierre Bordieu, Cockerham considered lifestyles largely as an outcome of structural factors. In this particular case, this *habitus* was affecting mostly working-class males, primarily manual workers, who died most frequently because CVD in middle age:

> Policy, societal stress, and health lifestyles appear to be the major potential sources of adverse male health in the region and each is found to make an important contribution to rising male mortality. But, ultimately (...) negative health lifestyles are the primary social determinant of the decline in life expectancy. The structure surrounding the daily life of middle-aged working-class males both limited and shaped choices to the extent that their lifestyle led to early deaths. This development was bound up in the larger structure of socialist societies, with their centralized planning and control systems that determined the opportunities and quality of life for their citizens. The needs of the state came first

---

22 Galea (2007), and Berkman et al. (2014) do not even mention the issue while Kunitz (2006), a remarkable book in many aspects, dedicates about a page to discussing the evolution of health during the transition to a market economy in Eastern Europe and the republics of the former Yugoslavia.

23 Cockerham (1999), *Health and social change*, ix, 1.

and the state never reached a position of improving the life of the individual; rather, the party elite was able to corrupt the system for their own ends, while the average person in a European socialist country fared poorly, not only in material goods and health, but in personal freedom and initiative.[24]

Levels of LEB in the Eastern European countries in the mid-1960s equaled or exceeded those in the West, but then adult mortality started to increase and by the early 1970s, LEB for Soviet men was decreasing, and the same happened in Bulgaria, Czechoslovakia, Hungary, Poland, and Romania.

> Something was causing mortality to rise in these countries and it was not clear what. As this development continued, an obviously embarrassing trend for socialism was emerging. The Soviet Union responded by not publishing figures on life expectancy after 1972 and on infant mortality after 1974.[25]

Since the 1960s, in all the countries of the Soviet bloc there were major increases in the frequency of smoking and alcoholic beverage consumption, and the predominant diet was notably unhealthy — with a high content in carbohydrates, saturated fat, scarcity of fresh produce and fruits, and lack of variety of food; furthermore, physical exercise was mostly missing for the population at large.[26] On this background, the sudden transition to a market economy elicited major changes that presumably could have a harmful effect on health. In Russia, said Cockerham, the strongest stressor appeared to be the loss of security as the guaranteed jobs and price controls of communism disappeared and low wages and pensions made life extremely difficult in a context of increasing cost of living. "Stress may have been most severe for middle-aged working-class males tasked with being their family's main provider".[27] This can be part of the explanation that the mortality rate for Russian men aged 40 to 49 which was 9.2 deaths per 1,000 in 1990, one year before the end of the USSR, jumped to 16.3 — an increase of 77% — in 1995. For most Russians, life became particularly hard since the end of the Soviet Union. It was estimated that over one-third of the population, some 44 million out of 148 million, were living below the poverty line in 1998.[28] Cockerham cited Canadian sociologist Robert Brym who pointed out that in 1991, the last year of the USSR, the richest 10%

---

24 Cockerham, *Health and social change,* 52, 251.
25 Cockerham, *Health and social change,* 9.
26 Cockerham, *Health and social change,* Ch. 2.
27 Cockerham, *Health and social change,* 106.
28 Cockerham, *Health and social change,* 97, 100.

of all Russians earned 4.5 times more than the poorest 10%, while by 1994, this ratio had jumped to 15 times more. Thus, in few years Russia became one of the most inegalitarian countries in the world with respect to income.[29] On the other hand, while 53% of the Russian population reported to smoke in 1985, about 67% did in 1992, which represented a significant increase, to some extent connected with the successful targeting of Russians as a vast, relatively new market, by Western tobacco companies.[30]

In other countries of Eastern Europe similar factors would be operating. For instance, in Bulgaria the transition from a centrally planned to a market economy led to the abolition of food subsidies, a decline in agricultural production, a large inflation of food prices resulting in an increase in the proportion of income spent on food, significant increases in the rate of unemployment, a decrease in the real incomes of the population, particularly of pensioners, and a general decrease of social benefits, all of which led to higher risk of nutrient deficiencies and unhealthful diets among Bulgarians.[31]

As argued by Cockerham, it is impossible to deny the fact that the period of adjustment after the demise of the USSR was highly stressful for the Russian population. The notion of "shock" mortality would imply that the rapid and negative effects of the collapse of communism would have stimulated an increase in death rates. However, Cockerham asserted that while certainly the population was stressed and mortality from natural causes rose during the postcommunist period, it was not clear "how the 'shock' of the transition contributed to the death toll".[32]

Overall, Cockerham blames the mortality crisis of the countries of Eastern Europe and the old USSR to the lifestyles that had been favored by the political regimes in power and which to a considerable extent were strengthened by the sudden transformation of the centrally planned economies into free-market capitalism. The only mention to the potential health effects of the Chernobyl disaster in Cockerham's book is a sentence asserting that in Ukraine and Belarus the effects of radiation from the Chernobyl accident had not yet produced any significant increases in cancer rates, excepting "a slight upward trend in thyroid cancer in children"[33]

One year after Cockerham's book, the multiauthor volume titled *The mortality crisis in transitional economies* was published under the editorship of two

---

29 Cockerham, *Health and social change*, 96.
30 Cockerham, *Health and social change*, 113.
31 Cockerham, *Health and social change*, 225.
32 Cockerham, *Health and social change*, 105.
33 Cockerham, *Health and social change*, 26.

economists with connections to the United Nations, Giovanni Andrea Cornia and Renato Paniccià. Thirteen of the 17 chapters of the book referred to the mortality crisis in Eastern Europe and the old USSR, and despite being mostly descriptive, some of the chapters discussed the potential causes of the mortality crisis. Psychosocial stress, institutional changes, poverty, environmental degradation, and alcohol abuse appeared frequently cited in the book as major potential causes of the mortality crisis. In the first chapter of the book, Cornia and Panniccià discussed psychosocial stress as the key factor contributing to mortality, but concluded that considering the contributions of the volume, the transition's mortality crisis remained largely unexplained.[34]

In 2005, Elizabeth Brainerd and David Cutler examined the potential causes of the mortality crisis in the former USSR.[35] After a meticulous discussion of changes in health services, traditional risk factors for CVD (hypertension, cholesterol, diabetes, obesity, and smoking), diet, material deprivation, and psychosocial factors, Brainerd and Cutler concluded that they could explain about half of the increase in mortality. About half of that half would be due to alcohol abuse, so that about half of the excess mortality remained unexplained.

A few years later some epidemiologists pointed to a different factor as cause of the mortality crisis. The examination of data from Eastern Europe and the former USSR by a group of British researchers led by David Stuckler showed that mass privatization programs appeared associated with a short-term increase in adult mortality. The authors of this investigation interpreted that male unemployment – which was increased substantially by mass privatization – was an intermediate link in the causal chain.[36] For David Stuckler it was remarkable that Belarus, which had taken a more gradualist approach to the transition to a market economy and had privatized their state-controlled economies in stages, had seen much better health outcomes, while in nearby countries quick programs of privatizations and layoffs caused severe economic and social disruption.[37] Controversies followed in which initial enthusiasts of quick privatization, namely Jeffrey Sachs, claimed not to be responsible for what followed after those policies were implemented in the countries of the former Soviet bloc.[38] Whatever

---

34 Cornia & Paniccià (2000), *The mortality crisis*, 4.

35 Brainerd & Cutler (2005), "Autopsy on an empire: Understanding mortality in Russia and the former Soviet Union," *Journal of Economic Perspectives* 19(1), 107–130.

36 Stuckler, King & McKee (2009), "Mass privatization and the post-communist mortality crisis," *Lancet* 373, 399–407.

37 Stuckler & Basu (2013), "How austerity kills," *The New York Times*, May 13, A19.

38 Sachs (2009), " 'Shock therapy' had no adverse effect on life expectancy in Eastern Europe," *Financial Times*, Jan 19; Anonymous (2009), "Ex-communist reform: Mass murder and the marthe case, what is now undeniable is that in the context of the countries in which a market economy replaced the formerly planned economy, Belarus had a miserable performance in terms of duration and depth of the mortality crisis (Tab. 1.1).

Over time and perhaps in part because of the incorporation of many countries of Eastern and Central Europe that had been part of the Soviet bloc into the European Union, the mortality crisis of the transition was increasingly thought of as something pertaining to the old Soviet Union or even just Russia. In 2013 Johan Mackenbach argued that the setting up of more or less democratic governments and market economies in the 1990s in the Western Balkans, Central and Eastern Europe and the former USSR implied painful economic adaptations and disruptive changes resulting in life expectancy declines in many countries. "But some countries emerged quickly from this painful phase with a renewed increase of life expectancy." For Mackenbach this was applicable for instance to the Baltic nations.[39] However, as we have seen, for Estonia, Latvia, and Lithuania the mortality crisis was acute and protracted, lasting over two decades (Tab. 1.1).

Alcohol and the mortality crisis

In a 2013 paper, Jay Bhattacharya, Christina Gathmann, and Grant Miller, economists working on health issues, rejected the view that the sudden privatization of the formerly planned economies was a major factor in the excess mortality of the countries of the former Soviet Union.[40] Analyzing alcohol consumption and crude death rates for the Russian *oblasts* (administrative units), Bhattacharya et al. found that the surge in deaths between 1990 and 1994 "occurred primarily among alcohol-related causes and among working-age men (the heaviest drinkers)", and argued that the key factor in explaining the increase in mortality was the end in 1988 of the Gorbachev anti-alcohol campaign, that had started in 1985. The end of that campaign "explains a large share of the mortality crisis," said Bhattacharya et al., who concluded that "Russia's transition to capitalism and democracy per se was not as lethal as often suggested."

———
ket," *The Economist*, Jan 22; David Stuckler and his coauthors also contributed to this controversy, see cited references.

39 Mackenbach (2013), "Political conditions and life expectancy in Europe, 1900–2008," *Social Science & Medicine* 82, 134–146.

40 Bhattacharya et al. (2013), "The Gorbachev anti-alcohol campaign and Russia's mortality crisis", *American Economic Journal — Applied Economics* 5(2), 232–260.

It is obvious that alcohol abuse and alcoholism, as other forms of substance abuse, played a role, particularly in Russia and probably also in other countries of the old Soviet Union. It has been often said that many frustrations of life under the forced "happiness", political repression and relative material scarcity prevailing in the countries of the Soviet bloc expressed themselves in alcohol abuse, which has deep roots and a long history among Russian males. Alcoholic beverages were recognized as an excellent source of revenue by Russian rulers since the times of Ivan the Terrible. By 1860, vodka, the national drink, was the source of 40% of the government's revenue.[41] "The greatest pleasure of this people is drunkenness, in other words, oblivion. Poor folk! they must dream to be happy". This was the view of the Marquis de Custine, a 19th-century French aristocrat whose observations on Russia look relevant two centuries later.[42] But the issue of alcohol is not exclusively Russian. Worldwide alcoholism is a major problem, but as a public health problem it is especially severe in Europe, and particularly in Eastern Europe. According to 2014 WHO data, Belarus, with an annual consumption of 17.6 litres of pure alcohol per capita was the European country of Europe with the highest alcohol consumption, followed by Moldova (16.8 litres), Lithuania (15.5), Russia (15.1), Romania (14.4), Ukraine (13.9), Andorra (13.8), Hungary (13.3), Czechia and Slovakia (both 13.0). These are all countries that were hit by the transitional mortality crisis. At lower levels of alcohol consumption per capita in Europe are Portugal (12.9), Poland (12.5), Servia (12.6), Finland and Latvia (12.3), France & Croatia (12.2), and Ireland (11.9), as well as countries like Britain (11.6), Spain (11.2) or Italy (7.6), often considered as heavy drinkers.[43]

In April 1982, the prices of vodka and most other alcoholic beverages were increased in the USSR, with the minimum price of vodka rising by 50%. The same year, LEB for Russian males increased by six months. The anti-alcohol campaign of Gorbachev is generally agreed to have been far more effective than previous efforts by the Soviet government to reduce alcohol consumption. The campaign included administrative measures, such as rationing (e.g., one bottle of vodka per adult per month), restricted hours of sale of alcohol, detention of publicly intoxicated individuals in a drunk tank, and an absolute ban of alcohol consumption in public places and institutions.[44] The campaign coincid-

---

41 Suddath (2010), "A brief history of Russians and vodka", *Time* January 5.
42 Booth (2020), "Astonishing drinking sessions and epic hangovers in the world's booziest nation", *The Telegraph* January 28.
43 WHO (2018), *Global status report on alcohol and health 2018.*
44 Grigoriev & Andreev (2015), "The huge reduction in adult male mortality in Belarus and Russia: is it attributable to anti-alcohol measures?", *PLoS ONE* 10(9), e0138021.

ed with a rapid reduction of mortality, especially of adult males, but did not have long-term effects. In 1988 the campaign was terminated — that year, tax revenues from sales of vodka accounted for 35% of the Soviet budget.[45]

It seems well proven that in Russia and Belarus alcohol consumption strongly decreased for a few years since 1985, but in the late 1980s started increasing, with major increases after 1989 and a steady rising trend that extends to the 2010s, when alcohol consumption per capita in both countries was at levels about 50% higher than in the highest consumption period of the USSR in the early 1980s.[46] In the 1990s, immediately following the dissolution of the USSR, there were basically no antialcohol policies in the new independent republics, and their governments were almost powerless to control the production and circulation of alcoholic beverages. Imports largely increased and competition led the prices of alcoholic beverages to historic lows. These factors contributed to a sharp rise in alcohol consumption. The situation could have been particularly severe in Russia, where the state alcohol monopoly was abolished in 1991 and a portion of the alcohol industry was privatized.[47]

That alcoholism and alcohol abuse had a role in the mortality crisis of the 1990s in the former republics of the USSR seems quite obvious just by noticing the major increases of mortality of Russian males because liver cirrhosis, suicides, homicides or accidents, all of them causes of death very often connected with episodes of drunkenness. The increases of CVD mortality of Russian men in the 1990s can be to a large extent attributed to alcohol consumption. Now, is that a reason to deny the role of economic, political, social and cultural factors in these deaths? Alcohol consumption is often a mechanism to deal with personal frustration, which in turn is very often linked to social and economic processes.[48] This, which has been often emphasized in relation to the so-called deaths of despair in the US, looks obviously applicable to a variety of national environments.

The debate on the role of alcohol consumption versus the influence of socioeconomic factors as well as other controversies on the cause or causes of the mortality crisis in Eastern Europe never were very visible, but they have not ended. Un 2013, from an anthropological perspective, Michelle Parsons empha-

45 Cockerham (1999), *Health and social change*, 50.
46 Grigoriev & Andreev (2015), "The huge reduction", Figure 1.
47 Andreev et al. (2013), "Comparing alcohol mortality in Tsarist and contemporary Russia: Is the current situation historically unique?", *Alcohol & Alcoholism* 48(2), 215–221.
48 Case & Deaton (2015), "Rising morbidity and mortality in midlife among white non-Hispanic Americans in the 21st century", *PNAS* 112(49), 15078–15083; Sterling & Platt (2022), "Why deaths of despair are increasing in the US and not other industrial nations — Insights from neuroscience and anthropology", *JAMA Psychiatry*, February 2.

sized in her survey of the mortality crisis in Russia that after the demise of the USSR "the majority of the Russian population found themselves living in poverty (...), almost everyone lost something in the early 1990s and all Russians were "losers", at least momentarily".[49] Parsons concluded in her book that the excess mortality "was but the biological end-point of political-economic processes that have psychosocial consequences". Consistent with this point of view, the perspective that attributes a major role in the mortality crisis to privatization factors has received new support from an investigation that found that mortality rose significantly faster in cities of the European part of Russia in which privatization took place quickly.[50]

A chronology

Something that apparently is often overlooked when discussing the mortality crisis in the old Soviet bloc is the concrete chronology of the events, which can be summarized as follows.

- *1985, March*, Mikhail Gorbachev assumes the general secretariat of the Central Committee of the Communist Party of the Soviet Union (CPSU), starting the period of *glasnost* (transparency) and *perestroika* (restructuring), as well as the anti-alcoholism campaign.
- *1986, April 26*, explosion of reactor No. 4 of the Chernobyl nuclear power plant, located in Ukraine, 17 km from the border with Belarus.
- *1988, October*, official termination of the anti-alcoholism campaign in the USSR.
- *1989*, in January the Soviet withdrawal from Afghanistan concludes; in Poland, Hungary, Czechoslovakia, Bulgaria, and East Germany, communist parties in office are forced to weaken political control, a transition to a parliamentary democracy starts; in Romania, Nicolae Ceaușescu, general secretary of the Communist Party, and his wife Elena are executed on December 25 after their government fails in repressing mass demonstrations militarily.
- 1990, in August, West Germany and East Germany agree to unify and in September East Germany ceases existing as a political entity; fast privatizations start to remove the centrally planned economies all around Eastern Europe.

---

49 Parsons (2014), *Dying unneeded*, 174–175.
50 Azarova et al. 2017, "The effect of rapid privatisation on mortality in mono-industrial towns in post-soviet Russia: A retrospective cohort study," *Lancet Public Health* 2(5), e231-e238.

- *1991, March 17,* Union Referendum in the USSR, 78% of Soviet citizens answered "Yes" to the question "Do you consider it necessary to preserve the Union of Soviet Socialist Republics as a renewed federation of equal sovereign republics in which the rights and freedom of an individual of any nationality will be fully guaranteed?"
- *1991, August,* an attempted coup by the conservatives of the CPSU against Gorbachev failed; President of the Russian Federation Boris Yeltsin lead the response and dissolved the CPSU.
- *1991, December,* the Treaty of Belavezha signed by the presidents of Russia (Yeltsin), Ukraine (Kravchuk) and Belarus (Shushkiévich) declared the dissolution of the USSR; Gorbachev resigned, and the USSR ceased to exist.[51]

This chronological scheme is key for the comprehension of the potential links between Chernobyl and the mortality crisis. So much so because, surprisingly, in the investigations and controversies on the mortality crisis in Eastern Europe and the former USSR, the topic of Chernobyl has been remarkably absent. However, as it will be seen in the following chapters, the evolution of death rates and birth rates and sex ratios in the countries most affected by the Chernobyl disaster is remarkably consistent with an effect of the fallout on those indicators. It is undeniable that the misery, the psychosocial stress, the alcoholism, and the alcohol acute intoxications that afflicted the countries of the old Soviet bloc in the early 1990s must have had a causal role in the skyrocketing mortality that was observed at the time. The mortality crisis was for sure a multicausal phenomenon, but the way demographic rates and ratios evolved suggests that the fallout of the Chernobyl nuclear disaster may have been one of its contributing causes.

---

51 "Technically, the USSR ceased to exist on December 8, 1991. On that day the presidents of the three main European republics met stealthily in Belaveza, a secluded hunting lodge in the forests of Belarus. There they declared the USSR legally dissolved (...) Why did they do that? The answer is as simple as it is banal: for a question of power. Three brothers, Russia, Ukraine and Belarus killed the mother to keep the inheritance" (Rafael Poch, "La disolución de la URSS," *La Vanguardia* (Barcelona), December 6, 2017, my translation from Spanish into English, JAT).

Chapter 2
Chernobyl — The nuclear disaster

Chernobyl and the 2011 Fukushima Daiichi nuclear disaster in Japan are the two nuclear energy disasters rated at level 7, meaning maximum severity, in the International Nuclear Event Scale, but Chernobyl is generally considered the worst nuclear disaster in history. While the radioactivity released by the Fukushima disaster went mostly to the Pacific Ocean, Chernobyl released a greater amount of radioactivity which deposited on populated areas of Europe, though it also reached other continents.

April 25, 1986 — The Chernobyl explosions and the fallout

The now partially abandoned city of Chernobyl, in Northern Ukraine, is about 90 km north of the Ukrainian capital, Kiev, 160 km southwest of the Belarusian city of Gomel, and 20 km South the Belarussian border. The construction of the Chernobyl Nuclear Power Plant and the city of Pripyat to house the personnel of the plant began in the 1970s. In 1977 the first reactor was completed, and reactors number 2, 3 and 4 followed in 1978, 1981, and 1983, respectively. On April 26, 1986, in the process of testing problems of reactor number 4, two explosions of debated nature occurred at 01.23.40 a.m. with an interval of about two seconds. The reactor core was destroyed, and an open-air fire of the graphite used as moderator of the nuclear reactor followed, with three further explosions around 9:00 p.m.[1] The explosions and the temperatures of up to 5000 °C generated by the fire, that lasted until May 4, vaporized or converted into particulate matter that lofted several kilometers high into the atmosphere an unknown proportion, perhaps a third of almost 200 metric tons of uranium dioxide fuel and fission products. Radioactive gasses, iodine-131, cesium-137, strontium and plutonium radioisotopes, and other radioactive materials were released to the atmosphere.

The radioactive plume moved northwest towards Scandinavia, west toward the British Isles, southwest to Switzerland and Italy, and south and east to the Black Sea region and the Middle East. Reports from China, Japan, and the United States indicated that within one week radioactivity had reached the entire north-

---

1 De Geer et al. (2018), "A nuclear jet at Chernobyl around 21:23:45 UTC on April 25, 1986," *Nuclear Technology* 201(1), 11–22; Fabrikant (1987), "The Chernobyl disaster: An international perspective," *Industrial Crisis Quarterly* 1(4), 2–12; Plokhy (2019), "The Chernobyl cover-up: How officials botched evacuating an irradiated city".

https://doi.org/10.1515/9783110761788-006

ern hemisphere.[2] Over 200,000 square km, about the size of the United Kingdom, were significantly contaminated, with one quarter of this surface corresponding to areas beyond the borders of the USSR.[3] According to UNSCEAR, the specialized agency of the UN on atomic radiation, iodine-131 and cesium-137 were responsible for most of the radiation exposure received by the general population.[4] The ability of a radioactive substance to generate lasting harmful radioactivity depends on how fast its atoms disintegrate radioactively, which is measured by its half-life, the time that an initial amount decays to half because disintegration of its atoms. Plutonium radioisotopes have a half-life of tens or hundred years but were released in very small amounts. At the other estreme, radioactive gasses, iodine-131 and strontium-89 have a half-life of hours or days and they decay quickly.[5] Thus cesium-137, with a half-life of 30 years and released to the atmosphere in large quantities by the Chernobyl explosions and fires received initially most of attention as key component of lasting harmful radioactivity due to fallout. Radioactive iodine was later proven to have also had major effects.

Though many aspects related to the Chernobyl fallout are disputed, there is general agreement that the highest amounts of radioactive contamination fell on Russia, Belarus, and Ukraine, followed at a certain distance by other European countries.[6] According to a book published by the European Union, the ten countries which received the highest deposition of cesium-137 in Europe were Belarus (33.5% of the contamination deposited in Europe), Russia (23.9%), Ukraine (20%), Sweden (4.4%), Finland (4.3%), Bulgaria (2.8%), Austria (2.7%) Norway (2.3%), Romania (2.0%) and Germany (1.1%).[7] However, countries not included in this list like the United Kingdom, suffered significant radioactive contamina-

---

2 Fabrikant (1987), "The Chernobyl disaster: An international perspective," *Industrial Crisis Quarterly* 1(4), 2–12.
3 Chernobyl Forum (2006), *Chernobyl's legacy: Health, environmental and socio-economic impacts, and recommendations to the governments of Belarus, the Russian Federation and Ukraine.*
4 UNSCEAR (2000), "Sources and effects of ionizing radiation: UNSCEAR 2000 report to the General Assembly", II, 47.
5 IAEA (2006), Environmental consequences of the Chernobyl accident and their remediation: Twenty years of experience – Report of the Chernobyl Forum expert group 'Environment', Table 3.1, 19.
6 IAEA (2006), 314–315; Marples 1996, "The decade of despair," *Bulletin of the Atomic Scientists* 52(3), 20–31; Fairlie & Sumner (2006), "The other report on Chernobyl (TORCH) – An independent scientific evaluation of the health-related effects of the Chernobyl nuclear disaster with critical analyses of recent IAEA/WHO reports"
7 Izrael et al. (1996), "The atlas of caesium-137 contamination of Europe after the Chernobyl accident," in *The radiological consequences of the Chernobyl accident,* ed by Karaoglou et al., 1–10.

tion, and large areas of Asian Russia, East and Central China, and the Asian part of Turkey were highly contaminated.[8] An early report of the US Department of Energy estimated that about a third of the cesium-137 released at Chernobyl was deposited in Belarus, Ukraine and Russia, other third in the rest of Europe and other third out of Europe.[9] In 1988 the total radioactive cesium-137 released by Chernobyl was estimated as 70 PBq,[10] of which about 42% had been deposited within the USSR, 37% in Europe, 6% in the oceans and the remainder in the other regions of the northern hemisphere.[11] This estimate of 70 PBq was revised up in later years. Thus in 2006 the IAEA reported that an early estimate of the amount of cesium-137 released by the accident

> and deposited in the former USSR was made based on an airborne radiometric measurement of the contaminated parts of the former USSR; this estimate indicated that about 40 PBq (...) was deposited. Estimates of the releases have been refined over the years, and the current estimate of the total amount of cesium-137 deposited in the former USSR is about twice the earlier estimate (i.e. 80 PBq).[12]

On the basis of previous estimates in several sources it can be assumed that the amount of cessium-137 radioactivity deposited in the territory of the former USSR would be between a third and a half the total radioactivity deposited worldwide because of Chernobyl. If the USSR portion was 80 PBq, the world total would be well over 150 PBq. However, the same IAEA report estimated a world total of cessium-137 radioactivity of just 85 PBq.[13]

The aftermath

For several days the government of the USSR tried to cover up the disaster. On 28 April, two days after the explosions at Chernobyl, workers at the Forsmark nucle-

---

8 Macalister & Carter (2009), "Britain's farmers still restricted by Chernobyl nuclear fallout," *The Guardian* May 13; Yablokov & Nesterenko (2009), "Chernobyl contamination through time and space", *Annals of the New York Academy of Sciences* 1181, 4–30, 14.
9 Goldman et al. (1987), "Health and environmental consequences of the Chernobyl nuclear power plant accident."
10 PBq is the abbreviation of petabecquerel, a unit of radioactivity equal to a quadrillion (10^{15}) becquerels. The becquerel (Bq) is the radioactive activity of a material in which one nucleus disintegrates per second.
11 UNSCEAR (1988), 342.
12 IAEA (2006), 18.
13 IAEA (2006), 19, Table 3.1

ar power plant in Sweden, about 1100 km from Chernobyl, were found to have radioactive particles on their clothing that could not be attributed to any malfunction in their nuclear plant.[14] That day, the Swedish government contacted the USSR government to inquire about whether there had been a nuclear accident in the USSR, and the Soviet government denied it. It was only after the Swedish government suggested they were about to file an official alert with the IAEA, and reports on abnormal levels of radioactivity were released by Sweden, Norway, and Finland that the Soviet government admitted an accident had occurred.[15]

Two workers of the Chernobyl nuclear plant died in the explosion and 134 firemen and personal involved in the immediate emergency response were hospitalized with acute radiation syndrome, of which 28 died in weeks and 14 suspected radiation-induced cancer deaths followed within the next 10 years. Evacuation started even before the USSR government reported the explosion. Until the summer of 1986, well over 100,000 people were evacuated from highly contaminated areas, including all inhabitants of Pripyat, located 3 km from the nuclear plant — about 50,000 people. Another 230,000 people were relocated in subsequent years.[16] Several hundred thousand soldiers and workers of all republics of the USSR were sent to the area of the disaster to "liquidate" its consequences. The total number of "liquidators," as these clean-up workers were called, has been estimated to reach as many as 600,000, perhaps 800,000. They participated in the removal of radioactive detritus, surface land, trees, and all kind of contaminated materials from the areas surrounding the destroyed reactor. They also built a sarcophagus to cover the destroyed reactor.

Ten years after the disaster, in a paper published by the *Bulletin of Atomic Scientists* the historian David Marples commented how Chernobyl had been one of the most controversial industrial disasters of all times, with wildly exaggerated claims on its consequences and equally wild assertions dismissing its effects.

> The truth about Chernobyl has been bent from the start — the Soviet Union wanted to protect the reputation of its ambitious nuclear power program, and the nuclear industry everywhere wanted the public to believe that a similar disaster "could not happen here".[17]

---

14 Brown (2019), *Manual for survival – A Chernobyl guide to the future*; Schmemann (1986), "Soviet announces nuclear accident at electric plant," *New York Times*, April 29, A1.
15 Schmemann (1986), "Soviet announces nuclear accident"; Wikipedia, "Chernobyl disaster".
16 Chernobyl Forum (2006), "Chernobyl's legacy".
17 Marples (1996).

The severity of the radioactive contamination produced by the Chernobyl disaster was rarely quantified by specialized agencies in terms understandable to the public. When an attempt was made, it often came from nonspecialized sources. Specialized agencies such as IAEA and UNSCEAR had obvious conflicts of interest when generating assessments of severity because they have the promotion of nuclear power for peaceful purposes as an institutional established purpose. Despite the general agreement that probably more than half of the radioactive depositions caused by the Chernobyl disaster fell on countries other than Belarus, Ukraine and Russia, both UNSCEAR and IAEA were reluctant to produce estimates of the amount of radioactivity that affected countries that were not part of the Soviet Union. After the Chernobyl disaster, the USSR authorities classified the areas with level of radioactivity over 555 kBq/m^2 as areas of "strict radiation control" while areas below that level and over 37 kBq/m^2 were classified as "contaminated".[18] In its 2000 report, UNSCEAR estimated that besides zones in Belarus, Ukraine and Russia, there were other areas in Europe where the cesium-137 deposition density exceeded 37 kBq/m^2, notably in Finland, Norway, Sweden, Austria and Bulgaria, countries in which the cesium-137 deposition density did not exceed 185 kBq/m^2 except in localized areas, for example, a 2–4 km^2 area in Sweden and some mountainous areas in the Austrian Province of Salzburg.[19] A paper published in 1990 quantified the radioactive fallout from Chernobyl as causing an increase in radiation dose of 20% to 110% over the normal environmental burden to the inhabitants of Salzburg City in Austria, at a distance of about 1300 km from Chernobyl.[20]

The case of Bulgaria is particularly troublesome, as the scarcity of concrete information from specialized agencies makes difficult to assess reports that claim enormous levels of radioactive fallout after the Chernobyl disaster.[21] That is the case, for instance, of a website claiming, without reporting any scien-

---

18 Chernobyl Forum (2006), *Chernobyl's legacy: Health, environmental and socio-economic impacts, and recommendations to the governments of Belarus, the Russian federation and Ukraine*, 10.

19 UNSCEAR (2000), Annex J, 464.

20 Pohl-Rüling et al. (1990), The Chernobyl fallout in Salzburg, Austria, and its effect on blood chromosomes", *Acta Biologica Hungarica* 41(1–3), 215–222.

21 The map presenting estimates of the surface ground deposition of caesium-137 released in Europe after the Chernobyl accident in the 2000 report of UNSCEAR codes by color the deposition levels in all the European countries. The scale contains six colors, from light yellow (the least contaminated areas, levels of deposition below 2 kBq/m^2), to yellow, dark yellow, pink, dark pink, and red (the most contaminated areas, levels over 1489 kBq/m^2). The only countries that are blank on that map are the republics of the old Yugoslavia (except Croatia and Slovenia), Albania and Bulgaria. See Figure XI on page 464 of UNSCEAR (2000).

tific source, that after the formal end of the communist regime in Bulgaria, the Atomic Physics Department of Sofia University estimated that the total radioactivity registered in May 1986, following the Chernobyl disaster, was between 90 and 1,400 times higher than normal in Northern Bulgaria, 340 to 1,700 times higher than normal in Southern Bulgaria, and 1,300 to 31,000 times higher than normal in Bulgaria's mountain areas.[22] According to a Bulgarian online newspaper there were reports that between April 30 and May 2, 1986, radioactivity in Bulgaria was at 1000 times above normal.[23] However, these reports of such enormous levels of radioactivity in most of Bulgaria during the spring of 1986 following the Chernobyl disaster are not substantiated by a paper authored by researchers of the Faculty of Physics of the University of Sofia, which reported that at the time of Chernobyl, radioactivity in Bulgaria was monitored by five stations and in May 1986 at some of these stations the personnel started changing the filters every 6 hours when increased radioactivity was observed. The same source reports that the fallout of radioactive matter over Bulgaria was between 1.5 and 3.5 kg, which was estimated as amounting approximately to one thousandth of the radioactive matter deposited beyond the circle of 20 km around Chernobyl.[24] This technical information hardly interpretable for the lay public is not accompanied in the paper by any information on the levels of radioactivity registered in Bulgaria after the Chernobyl disaster. It is very likely the authors had that information. Where they perhaps trying to avoid creating turmoil in the country?

22 Dikov (2018), "How Bulgaria's communist regime hid the 1986 Chernobyl nuclear disaster from the public protecting only itself."
23 Sofia Globe staff (2020), "Bulgaria, April 1986: The Chernobyl cover-up", *The Sofia Globe*, April 26.
24 Vapirev et al. (1996), "Estimation of the total fallout of Sr-90 and Cs-137 over the territory of Bulgaria after the Chernobyl accident", *Bulgarian Journal of Physics* 23, 3/4, 129–147.

Chapter 3
Chernobyl and the timing of the mortality crisis

It has been often argued that Gorbachev's policies in the 1980s were a response to the political, social and economic decay of the USSR and the Soviet bloc at large. From that point of view, it would not be surprising to see unfavorable demographic trends during the period preceding the collapse of the USSR. For example, the dramatic decrease in birth rates observed in the late 1980s in many Soviet republics may have been more influenced by personal decisions around childbearing — in which hopelessness and lack of resources may have had a large role — and by long term demographic trends — largely related with the changes in women's position in society — than by any effect of radioactive fallout. As we will see, this reasoning may be plausible but may not fully explain the changes observed.

It is generally agreed that economic turmoil during the period in which the economic systems of the countries of the USSR and Eastern Europe were suddenly transformed into market economies very likely had adverse effects on mortality. During this transition, many ex-Soviet citizens became unemployed, and poverty and hopelessness became prevalent.[1] However, the effects of these socioeconomic and psychosocial factors could only occur after the Soviet Union broke up into 15 republics and after the economic meltdown was well underway, which did not occur until after the USSR ceased to exist at the end of 1991. It was indeed in January 1992 when Yegor Gaidar, President Yeltsin's Deputy Prime Minister, liberalized prices formerly under state control, with the expectation they would increase between three and five times. Over the next 10 months, however, prices rose by a factor of nearly 30, draining regular people's savings accounts, reducing the purchasing power of pensions and other fixed sources of income drastically, and causing widespread misery. At that time, in 1992, measures intended to quickly transform the state-owned economy into a privately owned collection of enterprises were set in place, launching a period of several years in which the Russian economy disintegrated.[2] But obviously, these events cannot explain mortality increases that were occurring as early as

---

1 Brainerd & Cutler (2005), "Autopsy on an empire: Understanding mortality in Russia and the former Soviet Union," *Journal of Economic Perspectives* 19(1), 107–130; Cornia & Paniccià (2000), *The mortality crisis in transitional economies.*
2 Satter (2017), *The less you know, the better you sleep: Russia's road to terror and dictatorship under Yeltsin and Putin.*

https://doi.org/10.1515/9783110761788-007

1987 in Belarus, Ukraine and Lithuania as shown by the drops in LEB observed in these republics (see Fig. 1.1, page 2).

Another explanation of the mortality crisis emphasizes the role of alcohol. According to Bhattacharya et al., the Gorbachev anti-alcohol campaign, unprecedented in scale and scope, and recognized by many as having been very effective in reducing alcohol consumption, began in 1985 and although it officially ended in October 1988, in practice it lasted beyond its official end, and the de facto end date of that campaign was 1991. [3] For these authors the campaign's end "explains a large share of the mortality crisis, implying that Russia's transition to capitalism and democracy was not as lethal as commonly suggested." Bhattacharya and coauthors use crude death rates for their analyses — which is less than ideal because crude death rates as health indicators are biased by population aging — and maintain that the Soviet republics in the West and in the Baltics exhibit *"mortality declines during the late 1980s* followed by similar surges during the early 1990s" (italics added), a pattern that would be "also present, but attenuated," in former Soviet republics with large Muslim populations for whom alcohol policy matters less. However, a further examination of the data (see Figs 1.1 and 1.2, pages 2 and 4, Tab 1.1 page 9) reveals that in Lithuania, Belarus, Ukraine, Kyrgyzstan and Kazakhstan, mortality started to increase and LEB started to decline in 1986, while in Russia, Latvia, and Armenia the same occurred in 1987 and in Estonia in 1988. Age-adjusted mortality rates shown in Figure 1B of the paper by Bhacharaya et al. also reveal that Russian mortality was increasing from 1986 to 1991. In Russia and all the aforementioned republics mortality continued rising and reached to a peak (a trough in LEB) around 1994. These data do not support the statement that Soviet republics in the West and in the Baltics exhibit "mortality declines during the late 1980s followed by similar surges during the early 1990s". Indeed, mortality was rising basically since 1986 at the time in which the anti-alcohol campaign was supposedly having its maximum effect.

Common explanations attributed rising male mortality in the countries of the old Soviet Union to psychosocial effects of the transition, or poverty, or a spike in alcohol abuse. Since psychosocial effects of the transition and generalized poverty did not occur before 1992 and abrupt increases in alcohol consumption very likely occurred after 1991 or at least 1988, these explanations are at odds with the fact that in Ukraine, Belarus, Lithuania, Kazakhstan, and Kyrgyzstan male mortality started to increase in 1987 — as male LEB peaked in 1986 — ,

---

3 Bhattacharya et al. (2013), "The Gorbachev anti-alcohol campaign and Russia's mortality crisis," *American Economic Journal – Applied Economics* 5(2), 232–260.

while in Russia, Latvia and Armenia male mortality started to increase in 1988 — as male LEB peaked in 1987 (Tab 1.1, page 9).

The chronology of the mortality crisis in Belarus, Ukraine and Lithuania is consistent with an effect of the Chernobyl disaster. The radioactive release occurred in the spring of 1986, mortality started to increase in 1987 in these three republics. Of them, Belarus and Ukraine were with Russia the three countries most contaminated by the Chernobyl fallout, while Lithuania also received considerable doses of radioactive fallout.[4] In addition to the radiation consequence of the disaster fallout, which obviously was more severe in the areas of Belarus, Ukraine and Russia surrounding the site of the disaster, hundreds of thousands of Soviet citizens, particularly males, were directly exposed to radiation when they were enrolled in the clean-up effort, they were the so-called liquidators, who were likely subjected to substantial radiation exposures. In the absence of other explanations for the mortality increase starting in 1987, the hypothesis that the mortality increase can relate to the Chernobyl disaster looks plausible and worth investigating.

----

4 Mastauskas et al. (1997), "Consequences of the Chernobyl accident in Lithuania," *IAEA Reports*.

Chapter 4
Birth rates and sex ratios after Chernobyl

In 1993, just seven years after the Chernobyl disaster, a paper by a large group of researchers led by V. I. Kulakov was published in *Environmental Health Perspectives*. The authors, clinical researchers affiliated with the All-Union Scientific-Research Centre for Maternal and Child Health Care in Moscow, had investigated the evolution of reproductive and perinatal disorders in two areas exposed to significant fallout from the Chernobyl disaster, the Chechersky district of the Gomel region in Belorussia, and the Polessky district of the Kiev region in Ukraine, each with a female population slightly over 11,000.[1] The paper reported that approximately 53% of the population in Polessky had lived in areas where the radioactive pollution of the soil after the Chernobyl disaster was greater than 20 kCi/km^2 (740 MBq/m^2), whereas only 20% of the population in Chechersky was exposed to this level of radioactive pollution, while most of the population in both areas, Chechersky and Polessky, lived in areas were soil pollution was reported by Kulakov et al. to be between 10 and 20 kCi/km^2, i.e., between 370 and 740 MBq/m^2. These numbers mean very little to anyone unfamiliar with radioactive contamination issues, but based on the information published in other sources, the levels of radiation cited by Kulakov et al. looked extremely high.[2] After the Chernobyl disaster Soviet authorities classified areas with more than 37 kBq/m^2 as "contaminated" while those over 555 kBq/m^2 were classified as areas of "strict radiation control".[3]

The study by Kulakov et al. included 688 pregnant women and their babies, and 7000 labor histories encompassing an 8-year period ranging from 3 years before the Chernobyl disaster in April 1986 to 5 years after it. In comparing birth rates before and after the nuclear accident, the authors found that the birth rate had significantly decreased from 17.1 to 14.4 per thousand population in Che-

---

1 Kulakov et al. (1993), "Female reproductive function in areas affected by radiation after the Chernobyl power station accident", *Environmental Health Perspectives* 101, 117–123.
2 kCi/km^2 means kilocuries per square kilometer, MBq/m^2 means megabecquerels per square meter. One becquerel (1 Bq) is the radioactivity implied by one radioactive disintegration per second, while a curie (1 Ci) corresponds to 3.7×10^{10} disintegrations per second, i.e., 3.7×10^{10} Bq. Since one kilocurie is one thousand curies (1 kCi= 1000 Ci), one megabecquerel is a million becquerels (1 MBq = 10^6 Bq), and there are 10^6 m^2 in 1 km^2, 1 kCi/km^2 = 37 MBq/m^2.
3 Chernobyl Forum (2006), *Chernobyl's legacy: Health, environmental and socio-economic impacts, and recommendations to the governments of Belarus, the Russian federation and Ukraine*, 10.

https://doi.org/10.1515/9783110761788-008

chersky, and from 17.0 to 11.2 in Polessky. The prevalence of extragenital disorders during pregnancy — mainly anemia, renal disorders, and hypertension — increased in the post disaster years from 23.1% in 1982 to 33.9% in 1990 in Chechersky and 7-fold, from 7.1% to 51.2%, in Polessky. The incidence of early toxemia increased by a factor of 2 to 3 in both districts, with the highest frequency in 1988–1989, and the risk of early and late spontaneous abortion increased by a factor of 2 to 2.5, though the rate of premature delivery remained substantially unaltered. Compared with the pre-Chernobyl period, in Chechersky perinatal mortality in the first 3 years after Chernobyl decreased from 11.5% to 7.3% due to a reduction in both fetal and neonatal deaths, while in Polessky it increased from 15.1% to 17.8%. In 1990 an increase in perinatal mortality was registered in both districts. The most frequent overall causes of perinatal mortality, both before and after the nuclear disaster, were asphyxia, congenital abnormalities, and respiratory distress but congenital abnormalities that remained the second most common cause of perinatal death increased by a factor of 2 after 1986. Always according to the report of Kulakov et al., the incidence of neonatal morbidity increased 3-fold in Polessky and 2-fold in Chechersky following the Chernobyl accident. In the context of increased rates of CVD and metabolic defects during the first year of age, high blood pressure (over 90–100 mm Hg) was found in 46% of the children examined in the post disaster years. Among the newborn the prevalence of illness increased by a factor of about 2.4 in both areas, with newborn suffering mostly somatic disorders (46%), hematological disorders (59%), and infectious diseases (16%). The authors of the investigation concluded that after the Chernobyl disaster pregnant women and their offspring revealed adaptational and pathological abnormalities of various organs and systems caused by radiation, which triggered a complex pattern of organic dysfunctions.

Four years after publication of the investigation by Kulakov et al., Denise Bard and other two authors affiliated with the Health Protection and Dosimetry Department of the Institute of Protection and Nuclear Safety at Fontenay-aux-Roses, Cedex, France, published a paper on the health consequences of Chernobyl.[4] The paper by Bard et al. examined what had been published in the ten years since Chernobyl about health consequences of the accident and concluded that except for increases in the incidence of childhood thyroid cancer, there was no evidence of any increase in health disorders that could be attributed to the Chernobyl disaster. Bard et al. had reviewed the investigation by Kula-

---

4 Bard et al. (1997), "Chernobyl, 10 years after: Health consequences", *Epidemiologic Reviews* 19(2), 187–204.

kov et al. and had found major flaws in it; for example, insufficient information on the methods, the maternal age distribution, and how subjects had been selected or congenital malformations had been ascertained. Bard et al. also found, "obvious errors in contamination units (kCi instead of Ci?)" in the Kulakov paper, so that "it is difficult to know exactly how contaminated these zones were." Furthermore, "since cumulative in utero doses over the entire pregnancy did not exceed 100 mSv for any of the exposed women, it is unlikely that even a properly designed epidemiologic study could show any excess risk for congenital malformations attributable to ionizing radiation alone." The study by Kulakov et al. had concluded that in the comparison before-after Chernobyl, miscellaneous pregnancy disorders had increased from 23.1% to 33.9% in the most contaminated district they had studied, and from 7.1% to 51.2% in the less contaminated zone, but considering the two districts "differed by a factor of 3 in their prevalence of these disorders before the accident, suggesting that the attention paid to these problems varied between the two zones", Bard et al. concluded that "more intensive screening since the accident may explain these increases." Regarding the increased incidence of toxemia and complications of labor in both districts reported by Kulakov et al., Bard et al concluded that the very brief description of methods made it "impossible to draw a conclusion about the reality of these results, especially since, to the best of our knowledge, similar facts have never been reported in connection with exposure to ionizing radiation." They also noted that in Belarus, Ukraine, and Russia birth rates "fell in the months following the accident nationally as well as in the contaminated zones", which was also true for numerous regions of the former USSR. Furthermore, the number of pregnancies "also decreased in Sweden, Norway, and Italy in the first years after the accident, but the "demonstration of a causal link with the accident is problematic" since these declines in the birth rate were not consistent with previous knowledge on the effects of ionizing radiation.

Overall, the article by Bard et al. discounted as mostly unsound — because improper reporting, inadequate methods, detection bias resulting from more intensive screening, and inconsistency with previous knowledge about biological effects of radiation — the information about reproductive and perinatal health disorders associated with the Chernobyl disaster reported by the Soviet team of Kulakov and colleagues. Previous knowledge, mostly based on studies of Japanese survivors of the atomic bombings of Hiroshima and Nagasaki, was not consistent with such effects for radiation doses around Chernobyl which, according to the estimates computed by relevant institutions, were very low. Therefore, "the demonstration of a causal link" was "problematic".

Leaving aside the theoretical considerations on the plausibility of a link between the Chernobyl nuclear accident and reproductive disorders, what is unde-

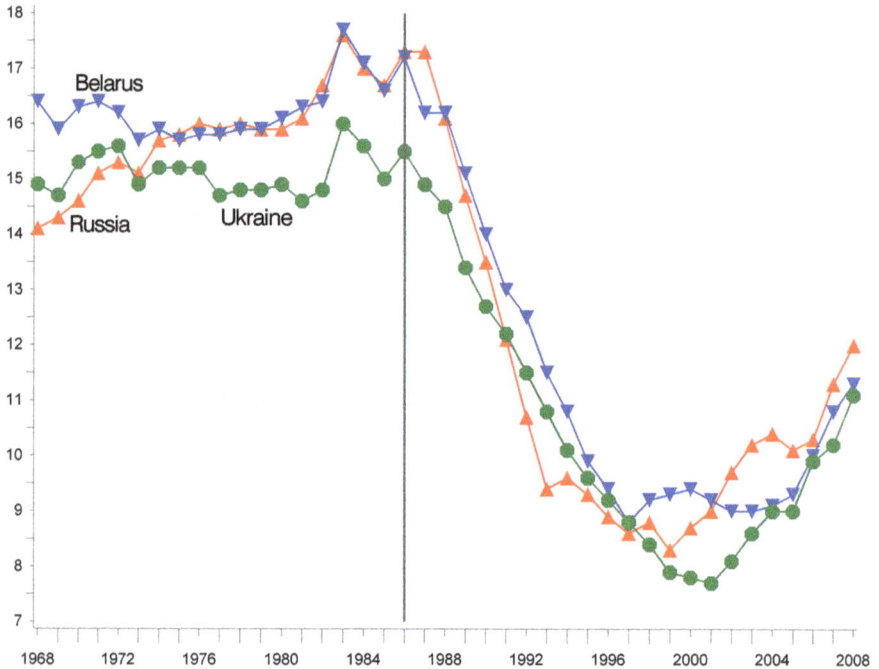

Fig. 4.1: Birth rate per 1000 population in Russia, Ukraine, and Belarus, 1968 – 2008. The vertical line marks the year of the Chernobyl disaster. Author's elaboration from data in the Human Mortality Database.

niable is that, after the Chernobyl disaster in 1986, birth rates significantly declined in Russia, Belarus, and Ukraine (Fig. 4.1), as well as in the Baltic nations (Fig. 4.2), and in the countries of Eastern and Central Europe (Fig. 4.3). However, the pattern of decline of birth rates in the countries of Eastern and Central Europe and in the Western Republics of the Soviet Union is remarkably different. In Poland, Hungary, Bulgaria and the two countries that at the time formed Czechoslovakia the decline of birth rates had started in the late 1970s or early 1980s, while in the Baltics, Russia, Belarus and Ukraine the birth rate decline started in the late 1980s. But the Baltics, Russia, Belarus and Ukraine were the republics of the USSR most affected by the Chernobyl fallout. Could this fall in birth rates during the late 1980s and the 1990s in the countries that had received the heaviest fallout from the Chernobyl disaster be a consequence of the exposure to radiation? The 2006 report of the Chernobyl Forum neither answered this question nor presented any data on birth rates nor cited published reports of reproductive and neonatal disorders. It stated, however, that

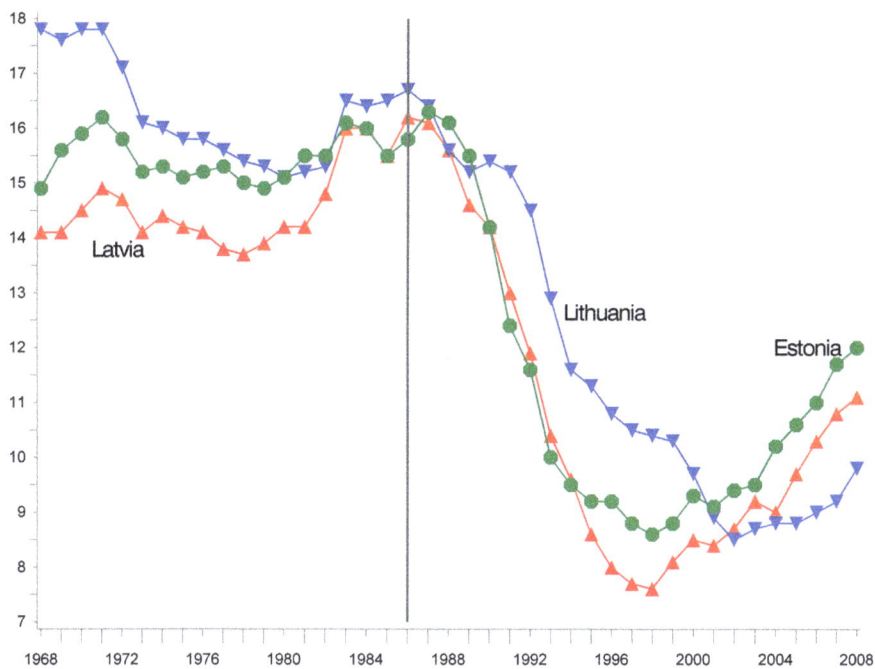

Fig. 4.2: Birth rate per 1000 population, Baltic nations, 1968 – 2008. The vertical line marks the year of the Chernobyl disaster. Author's elaboration from data in the Human Mortality Database.

> Because of the relatively low dose levels to which the populations of the Chernobyl affected regions were exposed, *there is no evidence or any likelihood of observing decreased fertility* among males or females in the general population as a direct result of radiation exposure. These doses are also unlikely to have any major effect on the number of stillbirths, adverse pregnancy outcomes or delivery complications or the overall health of children.[5]

The assertion that doses of radiation received by the population of the areas affected by the Chernobyl fallout were "low", was followed in the Chernobyl Forum report by the inference that there was neither evidence nor any likelihood of observing decreased fertility because of radiation exposure. The reasoning is fallacious, as the fact that radiation levels were low does not imply anything regarding the fertility levels observed. It does not matter that such low doses of radiation would be "unlikely" to have had any major effect on fertility rates or the number of stillbirths or adverse pregnancy outcomes.

5 Chernobyl Forum (2006), *Chernobyl's Legacy*, 19, italics added.

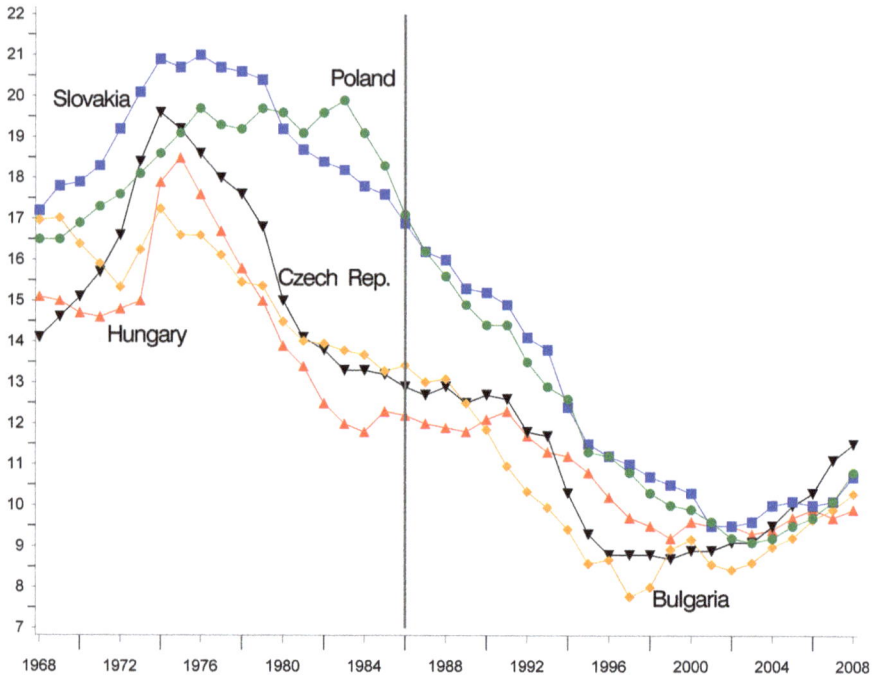

Fig. 4.3: Birth rate per 1000 population in five nations of Eastern Europe, 1968–2008. The vertical line marks the year of the Chernobyl disaster. Author's elaboration from data in the Human Mortality Database.

The view that doses of radiation as those received by the populations affected by the Chernobyl fallout could never be translated in any observable decrease in fertility was disputed in a report on the health consequences of the Chernobyl disaster authored by Russian, Belarusian, and Ukrainian authors that was published by the New York Academy of Sciences in 2009. That report stated that, since spontaneous abortions are not registered, a change in the abortion rate can only be inferred indirectly from a reduction in the birth rate.[6] As shown in Fig. 4.1, in Ukraine and Belarus the birth rate peaked in 1986 and declined steadily since that year. The same happened in Russia but with a delay of one year, as the Russian birth rate peaked in 1987. Also, as shown in Fig. 4.2, in the Baltic nations the birth rate that had been oscillating but overall, slightly increased in the twenty years before the Chernobyl disaster, had a precipitous drop after 1986. No

---

6 Nesterenko et al. (2009), "Consequences of the Chernobyl catastrophe for public health," *Annals of the New York Academy of Sciences*, 1181, 31–220, 192.

explanation has been given for this decline in the birth rate precisely after 1986 in the three countries that received the most severe fallout from the Chernobyl disaster, as well as in the Baltic states which after Belarus, Ukraine and the most western areas of Russia were the closest Soviet republics to the source of radioactive fallout.

It can be argued that the decline of birth rates in the countries of the Soviet bloc has its roots in social processes which have nothing to do with the Chernobyl disaster, i.e. the deterioration of social life that evolved toward the demise of communist-ruled political regimes around 1990. However, that notion looks a rather unlikely explanation for the decline of birth rates just after the Chernobyl disaster in Russia, Belarus, Ukraine, and the Baltics, where birth rates in the 1970s and the early 1980s had been either oscillating without a clear trend or rising. Certainly, the birth rate declines that started in the countries of the Soviet bloc in the late 1980s and continued during the 1990s and even extended to the early years of the 21st century can be largely explained by conscious decisions of men and women in reproductive age to delay or avoid conception, or to have an abortion. However, in the specific cases of Belarus, Ukraine, and Russia, as well as the Baltic nations, the chronology of the birth decline looks surprisingly consistent with being at least partly due to a higher frequency of spontaneous abortions related to the exposure to the Chernobyl fallout. That this is a hypothesis worth to be investigated is also supported by the fact that a sharp increase in the sex ratio at birth has been reported in the countries of Central and Eastern Europe following the Chernobyl disaster. The sex ratio at birth (males to females or males to all births) increases as an effect of exposure to ionizing radiation.[7] According to the data reported by Victor Grech, a Maltese pediatrician, comparing the years 1981-1985 and 1986-1990, the ratio males to total births had a post-Chernobyl increase of 3.1% in the Baltic States, 2.0% in the Russian Federation, and 2.1% in the area formed by Belarus, Ukraine and Moldova. Grech also reported a birth deficit in the post-Soviet states in the ten years following Chernobyl estimated in 2.07 million, of which 1.09 million would be accounted by Belarus and Ukraine alone. The evolution of both birth rates and sex ratios at birth after Chernobyl is therefore consistent with a plausible radiobiological effect of the Chernobyl disaster on fetuses and germ cells.

---

7 Grech (2014), "The Chernobyl accident, the male to female ratio at birth and birth rates", *Acta Medica* 57(2):62–67; Scherb & Voigt (2011), "The human sex odds at birth after the atmospheric atomic bomb tests, after Chernobyl, and in the vicinity of nuclear facilities", *Environmental Science and Pollution Research* 18:697–707; see also in the same journal (19:2456–2459 and 19:4234–4241) the critique by Bochud & Jung (2012), and the rebuttal by Scherb & Voigt (2012)-

Chapter 5
Soviet and post-Soviet cover-up

The fact that the Soviet government attempted to cover up the importance of the accident was obvious from the early days of the accident, when reports from Scandinavia forced the USSR government to acknowledge a major nuclear release. As Dr. Mikhail Balonov explained in a 2016 symposium on Chernobyl, reliable information about the accident and the resulting radioactive contamination was initially unavailable and the people residing in the affected areas, including the neighboring city of Pripyat, learned about the accident primarily through hearsay rather than from official government reports. This lack of communication likely contributed to the high levels of exposure of some nearby populations who did not have the information needed to take protective actions.[1] It is now uncontroversial that many million people were exposed to radiation, likely at doses much higher than has been reported. The Chernobyl Forum report did not provide any estimate of the total amount of radiation released by the explosions in reactor No. 4 of the Chernobyl nuclear plant, but according to Vassily B. Nesterenko of the Belorussian Institute of Radiation Safety (Minsk) and Alexey V. Yablokov of the Russian Academy of Sciences (Moscow), without taking the gaseous radionuclides into account, the release was "many hundreds of millions of curies, a quantity hundreds of times larger than the fallout from the atomic bombs dropped on Hiroshima and Nagasaki".[2] Information from other countries provides insights on the magnitude of the radioactive fallout generated by the Chernobyl disaster. Thus, in May 2009, 23 years after the Chernobyl accident, it was revealed by Dawn Primarolo, UK Minister of State for Public Health, that 369 farms and 190,000 sheep were still affected in the UK by radioactive pollution from Chernobyl. Minister Primarolo declared at the time that in 1986, approximately 9700 farms and 4.2 million sheep were put under restriction across the United Kingdom because of the Chernobyl radioactive fallout on Britain.[3] According to various reports, Sweden received around 4% or 5% of the cesium-137 thrown to the atmosphere by the explosions in reactor number 4 of the Cherno-

1 Samet et al. (2018), "Gilbert W. Beebe Symposium on 30 Years after the Chernobyl Accident: Current and Future Studies on Radiation Health Effects", *Radiation Research* 189, 1, 5–18.
2 Nesterenko & Yablokov (2009), "Chernobyl contamination: An overview", *Annals of the New York Academy of Sciences* 1181, 4–30.
3 Macalister & Carter (2009), "Britain's farmers still restricted by Chernobyl nuclear fallout", *The Guardian*, May 13.

https://doi.org/10.1515/9783110761788-009

byl power plant.[4] But cesium is absorbed by plants and mushrooms and concentrated in muscle tissue consumed as meat, and 30 years after the accident, the recommended exposure limit of cesium-137 was exceeded in berries, fish and game in Swedish areas that had received severe fallout.

While reports of governments and the Chernobyl Forum acknowledge the importance of early efforts to mitigate radioactive contamination by evacuating population and removing contaminated materials, these official reports never mention that government actions to mitigate the disaster were in many cases probably harmful and contributed to increase the level of exposure. Thus, there is massive "anecdotal evidence" that the work of the liquidators exposed several hundred thousand people, mostly males, from all republics of the USSR to high doses of radiation.[5] Furthermore, for the purpose of keeping radioactivity contained, the effort of the liquidators, despite their altruism and heroism, was probably useless to a large extent. During the chaotic period following the demise of the USSR the wood heavily contaminated with radioactive materials that had been buried under sand was removed from the ditches where it had been put. It disappeared and was probably used as firewood or sold by those who removed it; similarly, hundreds of heavily contaminated machines that had been abandoned by the liquidators in restricted zones were stolen and were likely resold wherever buyers could be found.[6]

In 1986, in the weeks after the April 26 Chernobyl explosions, several thousand buses were used for the evacuation of residents in contaminated areas. During the evacuation those buses became heavily contaminated by radioactive deposition, but then they were returned to use in public transportation in cities and towns mostly in Ukraine and Belarus, where they caused further exposure of the population to radiation.[7] As convincingly argued by Kate Brown, radioactive fallout contaminated vegetable produce, meat, milk, firewood, and leather from cattle to a much higher degree than accepted by governments and experts from UN agencies. While according to UNSCEAR the doses received by the liquidators who were exposed to high levels of external irradiation within days or weeks after the accident were estimated mainly from biological indicators because

---

4 Izrael et al. (2016), *The atlas of caesium-137 contamination of Europe after the Chernobyl accident*, European Union, Brussels; Alinaghizadeh et al. (2016), "Total cancer incidence in relation to ^{137}Cs fallout in the most contaminated counties in Sweden after the Chernobyl nuclear power plant accident: a register-based study", *BMJ Open* 6, 12, e011924.
5 Alexievich (2019), *Voices from Chernobyl*; Brown (2019), *Manual for survival: A Chernobyl guide to the future*.
6 Alexievich (2019), *Voices from Chernobyl*.
7 Plokhy (2019), "The Chernobyl cover-up: How officials botched evacuating an irradiated city".

"dosemeters (sic) were either not operational nor available",[8] there are witness accounts that many liquidators had dosimeters and even some of them had as their specific mission to examine the level of radiation with repeated measurements.[9] Attempts to cover up the fact that levels of radioactive exposure were much higher than usually acknowledged were likely behind three robberies that occurred in 1990 in the Institute of Radiation Medicine in Minsk, the Belarussian capital, and research institutions in Moscow, and in Bryansk, a city in western Russia. Computers, floppy disks and even notebooks containing thousands of data on radiation exposures were stolen in these robberies.[10] They were never recovered so that UNSCEAR and IAEA estimates of amounts of radiation were never based on primary data.

An obvious case of censoring to avoid inconvenient research and reports about the health consequences of the Chernobyl disaster was the incarceration in 2001 of the Belorussian pathologist Yury Bandazhevsky, who was director of the Medical Institute in Gomel, and the first to create an institute in Belarus dedicated to research on the Chernobyl disaster.[11] He and his wife Galina Bandazhevsky investigated how cesium-137 deposits in human organs and how the function of the cardiac muscle is altered by this radioisotope. In 1998, at the time when the Belorussian government launched plans to build the first Belorussian nuclear power plant, Bandazhevsky wrote a report to the government complaining of misuse of 17 billion rubles earmarked for Chernobyl research. A few months later he was arrested under a new antiterrorism law, tortured, and later sentenced with the institute's Deputy Director, Vladimir Ravkov, to eight years imprisonment on the grounds that he had received bribes. According to Amnesty International, Bandazhevsky's conviction "was widely believed to be related to his scientific research into the Chernobyl catastrophe and his open criticism of the official response to the Chernobyl nuclear reactor disaster on people living in the region of Gomel." He was released from prison in 2005, lived several years in Western Europe and then returned to do Chernobyl-related research in Belarus.[12]

The Soviet government first and the governments of Russia, Belarus and Ukraine later had strong interest in minimizing the Chernobyl issue. In addition,

---

8 UNSCEAR (2000), Vol. 2, 467.

9 Alexievich (2019). See for instance the sections titled "Soldiers' Chorus" and "People's Chorus". Overall, the word "dosimeter" appears 33 times in the book, which is a compilation of interviews with persons who witnessed the Chernobyl disaster or the work of the liquidators.

10 Brown (2019), 234.

11 Wikipedia, "Yury Bandazhevsky"; Brown (2019), 291–295, 308, 320.

12 Brown (2019), 314–317.

IAEA estimates of the radiation exposure that occurred as consequence of the Chernobyl disaster were the most optimistic, as expected from an agency committed to promotion of the use of atomic energy. Hence, it is hardly surprising that the Chernobyl Forum concluded that mostly low levels of radiation exposure had occurred. Since the estimated levels of radiation exposure were low, often claimed not to be much above natural background radioactivity, a natural conclusion based on previous studies of the Japanese A-bomb survivors is that such exposure could not be the cause of the high levels of disease and death observed immediately after Chernobyl. Therefore, the increased morbidity and mortality compared to pre-Chernobyl levels had to be attributed to psychological stress, to *radiophobia*. As stated in the report of the Chernobyl Forum, "the mental health impact of Chernobyl is the largest public health problem unleashed by the accident to date."[13]

---

13 *Chernobyl Forum: 2003–2005* (2006), 36.

Chapter 6
Effects of the radioactive fallout —
From early evaluations to the Chernobyl Forum

When days after the Chernobyl explosions it became obvious that it would be impossible to cover up the disaster, the strategy adopted by Soviet authorities — at the time of *glasnost* and *perestroika* which were generating many disagreements among them — was to minimize the importance of the disaster and the potential effects on health of the radioactive fallout. In that task the USSR had strong allies, as European governments were interested in assuring their populations that there were no major risks derived from the Chernobyl fallout, and all the major powers had vested interests in arguing that the low-dose radiation produced by either military or civilian uses of atomic energy was innocuous. By implementing actions such as the limited distribution of iodine to children and early evacuations and relocations of hundreds of thousand residents in the fallout areas, the Soviet government tried to assure the public that the health impact of the disaster would be minimal, in an effort to maintain its rapidly deteriorating credibility, which at the time, the last years of the USSR, was rapidly falling for many reasons.

Initial assessments of the impact of Chernobyl on health ranged in a wide zone of estimates. Three months after the Chernobyl disaster, John W. Gofman, a professor of molecular and cell biology at the University of California at Berkeley, predicted that Chernobyl would cause "475,000 fatal cancers plus about an equal number of additional non-fatal cases," occurring over time both inside and outside of the territory of the Soviet Union.[1] Gofman had degrees in chemistry and medicine, had worked for years in radiation research in connection with the Manhattan project and then in the Biomedical Research Division of the Livermore National Laboratory, where he had been an outstanding figure in investigations on the link between chromosomal abnormalities and cancer. Quite different was the assessment of Jacob Fabrikant, a radiologist who had been Chairman of the Public Health and Safety Task Force for the President's Commission on the Accident at Three Mile Island, who in 1987, just one year after the Chernobyl accident, argued that the health effects of the fallout would not be detectable beyond the borders of the USSR. However, he also noted that, though over a 30-

---

[1] Gofman (1990), "Assessing Chernobyl's cancer consequences: Application of four 'laws' of radiation carcinogenesis" (presented at the Symposium on Low-Level Radiation, National Meeting of the American Chemical Society, September 9, 1986).

https://doi.org/10.1515/9783110761788-010

year period, some 1500 added thyroid cancers could be expected as a result of the radioactive iodine deposited by the Chernobyl fallout.[2]

In 1990, four years after the Chernobyl accident, the US National Academy of Sciences published the BEIR V Report on effects of low-dose radiation. The report stated that for the Chernobyl accident,

> preliminary estimates suggest that up to 10,000 excess cancer deaths could occur over the next 70 years among the 75 million Soviet citizens exposed to the radioactivity released during the accident (...) among the 116,000 people evacuated from immediate high-exposure areas in the Ukraine and Byelorussia, there might be a detectable increase in the cases of leukemia and solid cancer.[3]

Five years after Chernobyl, in December 1991, the USSR ceased to exist, breaking down into 15 republics. In the largest one, the Russian Federation, under the presidency of Boris Yeltsin who had good relations with Western governments, the centrally planned economy was quickly transformed into a market economy through nationwide privatization of state-owned enterprises and liberalization of prices. In the ensuing economic collapse and inflation, a small number of oligarchs obtained a large share of the national property and wealth. At the same time, citizens of the ex-Soviet new republics, mostly males, were dying at much higher rates than when they were citizens of the USSR as a result of heart disease, liver cirrhosis, acute alcoholic intoxication, suicides, homicides, and other ailments. Given the broader context not much attention was paid to reports suggesting carcinogenic effects of the Chernobyl disaster in Europe,[4] reproductive disorders in women and increased morbidity in newborns, and higher than normal incidence of childhood cancer in parts of Belarus, Ukraine, and Russia where the fallout of Chernobyl had been particularly intense.[5]

In April 1996 over 800 experts from 71 countries met in Vienna, where the IAEA has its headquarters, at the international conference "One Decade After

---

2 Fabrikant (1987), "The Chernobyl disaster: An international perspective", *Industrial Crisis Quarterly* 1(4), 2–12.
3 National Research Council (1990), *Health effects of exposure to low levels of ionizing radiation: BEIR V.*
4 Michaelis et al. (1996), "Case control study of neuroblastoma in west-Germany after the Chernobyl accident", *Klinische Pädiatrie* 208, 4, 172–178; Petridou et al. (1994), "Trends and geographical distribution of childhood leukemia in Greece in relation to the Chernobyl accident", *Scandinavian Journal of Social Medicine* 22, 2, 127–131,E.; Petridou et al. (1997), "Infant leukaemia after in utero exposure to radiation from Chernobyl", *Nature* 387, 6630, 246.
5 Kulakov et al. (1993), "Female reproductive function in areas affected by radiation after the Chernobyl power station accident", *Environmental Health Perspectives* 101, 117–123; Stsjazhko et al. (1995), "Childhood thyroid cancer since accident at Chernobyl", *BMJ* 310(6982), 801.

Chernobyl" sponsored by IAEA, the European Commission, and WHO. The outcome was an IAEA report published soon after in several languages, including Russian, that summarized what according to IAEA had been learned after ten years of examining the consequences of the Chernobyl "accident" (the term was mentioned 34 times in the report) or Chernobyl "explosions" (2 times).[6] The term "disaster" now common in the literature referring to Chernobyl, did not appear in the brochure even once. In bulleted style the IAEA brochure listed facts related to the Chernobyl accident. It was stated that the accident had put 400 times more radioactive material into the atmosphere than the bomb dropped on Hiroshima; that atomic weapons tests in the 1950s and 1960s had put some 100 to 1000 times more radioactive material into the atmosphere than the Chernobyl accident; that many of the 600,000 to 800,000 liquidators received only low doses of radiation; that some 200,000 liquidators involved in the initial clean up received an average radiation close to 100 mSv, which is equivalent to about 1000 general chest X-rays, or about 5 times the maximum dose for workers in nuclear facilities (20 mSv per year); that average natural "background" radiation is 2.4 mSv/year; that in Belarus, where an estimated 70 % of the radioactivity was deposited, about 20 % of the population (2.2 million people) was in areas "where contamination initially exceeded (*sic*) 37 kBq/square meter — a low level not requiring decontamination and other control measures"; that outside of the former USSR, the highest national average radiation dose during the first year after the accident was 0.8 mSv, meaning an additional dose equal to about one third of the natural background radiation; and that a sharp increase in thyroid cancer among children, "the only major public health impact from radiation exposure documented to date," had been observed. The IAEA report, published as a brochure, also asserted that an increase in the incidence of thyroid cancer in adults who received radiation doses as children could occur, with the total number of cases possibly in the order of a few thousands; overall, other than thyroid cancer, long term health impacts from radiation had not been detected.

These reassuring messages contrasted however with the increasing frequency of reports of rising morbidity and mortality in the large areas where the Chernobyl fallout had fallen. Very soon, these health effects were attributed by the interested governments and international agencies to *radiophobia*. The rationale was that *the doses of radiation received by those getting ill or dying were too low to be causing those effect so soon*. However, the fallout from Chernobyl had likely been distributed very irregularly and could have been much higher in particular

---

6 IAEA (1996), *After Chernobyl: What Do We Really Know?*

locations as illustrated by observations in Sweden and Wales. In addition, the argument that the health effects of low radiation could not appear so soon was controversial in the scientific community[7] and was largely based on studies of Japanese A-bomb survivors who had suffered an acute exposure to a different form of ionizing radiation.

In 2003 eight agencies of the United Nations — AEA, FAO, OCHA, UNDP, UNEP, UNSCEAR, WHO, and the World Bank — and the governments of Belarus, Russia, and Ukraine, formed the Chernobyl Forum, which two years later, in 2005, released an assessment report titled *Chernobyl's Legacy: Health, Environmental and Socio-Economic Impacts*. A revised second edition of the report was released in 2006. The report claimed to be "the most comprehensive evaluation of the accident's consequences to date" and to represent "a consensus view of the eight organizations of the UN family according to their competences and of the three affected countries".[8] Concerning the health consequences of the disaster, the report stated that 28 emergency workers had died from acute radiation syndrome. However,

> So far, epidemiological studies of residents of contaminated areas in Belarus, Russia and Ukraine have not provided clear and convincing evidence for a radiation-induced increase in general population mortality, and in particular, for fatalities caused by leukaemia, solid cancers (other than thyroid cancer), and non-cancer diseases.
>
> However, among the more than 4000 thyroid cancer cases diagnosed in 1992–2002 in persons who were children or adolescents at the time of the accident, fifteen deaths related to the progression of the disease had been documented by 2002.

Regarding the number of deaths attributable to the Chernobyl accident, the report stated (italics added, JAT) that it had been claimed that

> tens or even hundreds of thousands of persons have died as a result of the accident. *These claims are highly exaggerated*. Confusion about the impact of Chernobyl on mortality has arisen owing to the fact that, in the years since 1986, thousands of emergency and recovery operation workers as well as people who lived in "contaminated" territories have died of *diverse natural causes that are not attributable to radiation*. However, widespread expectations of ill health and a tendency to attribute all health problems to exposure to radiation have led local residents to assume that Chernobyl-related fatalities were much higher.

---

7 Nussbaum & Kohnlein (1994), "Inconsistencies and open questions regarding low-dose health effects of ionizing radiation", *Environmental Health Perspectives* 102, 8, 656–667.

8 Chernobyl Forum (2006), *Chernobyl's Legacy*, 8. The following quotations of the report are from pages 14–16.

However,

> It is impossible to assess reliably, with any precision, numbers of fatal cancers caused by radiation exposure due to Chernobyl accident. Further, radiation-induced cancers are at present indistinguishable from those due to other causes.

Despite this stated impossibility of assessing reliably the number of fatalities due to the disaster, the executive summary of the report plainly stated that some 4000 deaths would be the total effect of the Chernobyl accident. This was based on estimates of cancer deaths among liquidators and residents in contaminated areas exposed to high levels of radiation. The full report stated nevertheless that among 6.8 million others living further from the explosion who received much lower doses, Chernobyl would kill about 5000, which would raise the projected death toll to 9000. This was not mentioned in the report's 50-page summary or the accompanying press release.[9]

The report stated that the highest radiation doses were received by emergency workers and on-site personnel. Among "more than 600,000 people [...] registered as emergency and recovery workers ('liquidators') [...] some received high doses of radiation" but "many of them and the majority of the residents of areas designated as 'contaminated' in Belarus, Russia and Ukraine (over 5 million people)" received radiation not much higher than doses due to natural background radiation. "It should be noted that early mitigation measures taken by the national authorities helped substantially to minimize the health consequences of the accident".[10]

On page 7 of the report, cases of thyroid cancer were mentioned as one of the main health impacts of the accident, mainly in children and adolescents at the time of the accident who drank milk with radioactive iodine and received high doses of radiation to the thyroid. "By 2002, more than 4000 thyroid cancer cases had been diagnosed in this group, and it is most likely that a large fraction of these thyroid cancers is attributable to radioiodine intake." On page 17 the number of cases of thyroid cancer observed in children of the three countries was said to be "close to 5000". It is explained however that the survival rate of these cancers is almost 99 % — though no timeframe for measuring survival is given. Apart from thyroid cancer in children the report stated that

---

9 Peplow (2006), "Counting the dead: 20 years after the worst nuclear accident in history, arguments over the death toll of Chernobyl are as politically charged as ever," *Nature* 440, 982–983.
10 Chernobyl Forum (2006), *Chernobyl's Legacy*, 17.

there is no clearly demonstrated increase in the incidence of solid cancers or leukaemia due to radiation in the most affected populations. There was, however, an increase in psychological problems among the affected population, compounded by insufficient communication about radiation effects and by the social disruption and economic depression that followed the break-up of the Soviet Union.[11]

The report acknowledged that radiation-induced increases in fatal leukemia, solid cancers and circulatory system diseases had been reported in Russian emergency and recovery operation workers, so that "in the cohort of 61,000 Russian workers exposed to an average dose of 107 mSv about 5% of all fatalities that occurred may have been due to radiation exposure." Note here that the number of fatalities which this 5% implies is not given and cannot be calculated because the total of fatalities at which this 5% applies is not provided. The report adds that these findings, "should be considered as preliminary and need confirmation in better-designed studies with individual dose reconstruction." On the other hand,

> The absence of a demonstrated increase in cancer risk — apart from thyroid cancer — is not proof that no increase has in fact occurred. Such an increase, however, is expected to be very difficult to identify in the absence of careful large-scale epidemiological studies with individual dose estimates.[12]

With respect to CVD,

> There appears to be some recent increase in morbidity and mortality of Russian emergency and recovery operation workers caused by circulatory system diseases. Incidence of circulatory system diseases should be interpreted with special care because of the possible indirect influence of confounding factors, such as stress and lifestyle.[13]

The report gave assurance that the main causes of death in the Chernobyl-affected region were "the same as those nationwide — CVD, injuries and poisonings — rather than any radiation-related illnesses" and remarked that "the mental health impact of Chernobyl is the largest public health problem unleashed by the accident to date."

In contrast to early estimates like that of the US National Research Council in 1990 of some 10,000 deaths as the long-term consequence of Chernobyl, and many people suspecting many more, the Chernobyl Forum press release reduced

---

11 Chernobyl Forum (2006), *Chernobyl's Legacy*, 7.
12 Chernobyl Forum (2006), *Chernobyl's Legacy*, 19.
13 Chernobyl Forum (2006), *Chernobyl's Legacy*, 19.

the death count to just 4000 fatalities. This was a bold move to pour water on the fire. For many scientists it was an obvious denial of the uncertainties resulting from limited data and a short period of follow up.[14]

---

14 Peplow (2006), "Counting the dead".

Chapter 7
Health effects of ionizing radiation —
How knowledge grew out of secrecy

Harmful properties of ionizing radiation or radioactivity, in the form of acute sunburnlike effects, were first identified soon after such radiation was discovered in the 1890s. In the early decades of the 20th century, radiation was found to cause skin cancer and leukemia was observed to be more common in radiologists. In 1928 the International Congress of Radiology formulated the first standards for radiation protection. At that time, it was widely believed among knowledgeable scientists that there was a threshold for the deleterious effects of radiation, that is, a dose below which there would be no damage.[1] These were very specialized matters, and the population at large was uninformed about such issues.

Radioactivity relates to phenomena occurring in the nuclei of atoms and scientists in the 1930s had the insight that bombs of huge power could be produced if the energy released by these nuclear phenomena could be triggered in some way. During World War II, under strict secrecy the governments of the UK, the US, and Germany invested resources into developing an atomic bomb. Only the US had the huge industrial resources sufficient to accomplish the task — the Manhattan project.

In the decades after the bombings of Hiroshima and Nagasaki, atomic bombs and nuclear energy were in the public eye and were the topic of much discussion. On August 6, 1945, an announcement from President Truman — who was at sea, returning from the Potsdam Conference — was filmed and then distributed to the press. The way Truman presented the news was as follows: "A short time ago, an American airplane dropped one bomb on Hiroshima, and destroyed its usefulness to the enemy...".[2] The press release distributed in Washington DC began in a slightly different way: "Sixteen hours ago, an American airplane dropped one bomb on Hiroshima, *an important Japanese Army base.* That bomb had more power than 20,000 tons of TNT [...] It is an atomic bomb. It is a harnessing of the basic power of the universe".[3] Three days later, on August 9, a second bomb was launched on Nagasaki. A major effort by the

---

1 Ad hoc Working Group, US Department of Health & Human Services (1985), *Report of the NIH ad hoc Working Group to develop radioepidemiological tables.*
2 Truman (2021), "President Harry Truman announces the Bombing of Hiroshima".
3 Lifton & Mitchell (1995), *Hiroshima in America: Fifty years of denial*, 4, italics added.

https://doi.org/10.1515/9783110761788-011

US government was to present the two bombs as directed against military targets and to reject the notion that they had caused any damage besides the thermal and mechanical effects of the explosion. There was no acknowledgement that other short or long-term consequences mediated by other effects of the bombs aside from their direct impacts could occur. General Leslie Groves, the military authority in charge of the Manhattan Project, rejected as Japanese propaganda the idea that survivors in Hiroshima and Nagasaki who had not been killed by the explosion were dying in great numbers following the bombings.[4] The deaths were attributed to delayed effects of burns.

Japan surrendered on August 15, and despite efforts of the US military to censor any information on deaths because of radiation, reports of unexplained deaths from the two bombed cities started to appear in newspapers. On August 29, Groves rebuffed the notion and declared emphatically that the atomic bomb was not an inhuman weapon.[5] The reality of deaths because of radioactivity had started to leak, though, raising concerns too about the Trinity test, the first atomic bomb that had been tested in Nevada in July 1945. The Pentagon's censorship office deleted about two thirds of a *Philadelphia Bulletin* article which reported that radioactivity from the Trinity test had spread to small towns in the surrounding region.[6]

The case had to be made vigorously that the atomic bomb tests had no consequences beyond the explosion itself. On September 9, Groves led a group of journalists to New Mexico's Alamogordo Bombing and Gunnery Range, where the Trinity test had been performed on 16 July 1945. Patrick Stout, a 29-year-old soldier who was General Groves' driver remained in the crater of the blast for several minutes, smiling and being photographed. Afterwards he was informed by one scientist that his exposure to radiation had been dangerous. Despite the PR narrative of no effects of atomic bombs except those immediately caused by the explosion, those working in the Manhattan Project and the top military knew about the acute and chronic effects of exposure to radiation. Twenty-two years later Patrick Stout was diagnosed with leukemia, the US army paid him "service-connected" disability, and he died at age 53.[7] Two physicists working in the Manhattan project, Harry Daghlian and Louis Slotin, died days after exposure to high levels of radiation because of accidents on August 21, 1945, and May 21, 1946. The cause of death was hidden by the military, attrib-

---

4 Lifton & Mitchell (1995), *Hiroshima*, 45.
5 Lifton & Mitchell (1995), *Hiroshima*, 46.
6 Lifton & Mitchell (1995), *Hiroshima*, 42.
7 Lifton & Mitchell (1995), *Hiroshima*, 52.

uted to "burns." Calculations showed that the radiation received by Slotin was equivalent to that received by Hiroshima residents one mile away from the hypocenter of the atomic bomb.[8]

In 1947 the US Atomic Energy Commission was established. The agency, which in subsequent decades would be known as the AEC, was created at the same time as the National Security Council and the Central Intelligence Agency (CIA), the three of them "national security bodies immune from democratic oversight".[9] The AEC formally transferred the control of atomic energy from military to civilian hands, though in truth, the AEC continued to have multiple links with the military.

Starting in 1946, the initial post-war US nuclear tests were conducted at remote locations in the Pacific Ocean, far from the US mainland. Then the first Soviet nuclear test took place in 1949 and the Cold War became full blown. The American monopoly on nuclear weapons had been lost, and the US government decided to significantly expand the development and production of nuclear weapons, which demanded repeated nuclear tests. Testing in the Pacific was cumbersome for many reasons and the Nevada Test Site was selected as the main location for subsequent tests. In January and February 1951, five air-dropped nuclear tests were conducted on Frenchman Flat, a dry lake at the Nevada Test Site. About 150 nuclear tests involving a total of 199 nuclear explosions were conducted there through 1963. Troops often participated, with little or no protection.[10]

In the early 1950s cattle and horses from ranches in the region surrounding the Nevada Test Site got burns that looked like those that had been noticed in cattle grazing at Chupadera Mesa, New Mexico, some 50 km away from the explosion site at Los Alamo, days after the Trinity test in 1945. The AEC had this information but did nothing to protect ranchers and residents in Nevada and Utah from the exposure to radiation resulting from the tests, though tests were announced in advance to the National Association of Photographic Manufacturers.[11] Between March and June 1953, 11 atomic tests took place on the Nevada

---

8 Lifton & Mitchell (1995), *Hiroshima*, 62–63.

9 Foner (2006), *Give me liberty!*, 781.

10 Comprehensive Nuclear-Test-Ban Treaty Organization (2022); Rice (2015), "Downwind of the atomic state: US continental atmospheric testing, radioactive fallout, and organizational deviance, 1951–1962", *Social Science History* 39, 647–676.

11 Blitz (2016), "When Kodak accidentally discovered A-Bomb testing: Two thousand miles away from the US A-bomb tests in 1945, something weird was happening to Kodak's film", *Popular Mechanics* June 20; Fradkin (1989), *Fallout: an American nuclear tragedy*, 105.

Test Site and some 5,000 sheep died across exposed areas of Utah and Nevada.[12] There was an outcry from ranchers, but the AEC claimed that the cause was probably eating poisonous plants. The Bordoli Ranch was 70 miles, about 115 km, from the Nevada Test Site. The Bordolis saw the bomb clouds passing over their ranch after the atomic tests. The three children in the family experienced skin reddening that was different from sunburns. Martin Bordoli had been born on December 1948. In 1955 he developed stem-cell leukemia, a rare disease that killed him ten months later. His doctor said the leukemia could be caused by the fallout, or perhaps by other things. The AEC repeatedly stated that levels of radioactivity resulting from nuclear tests were safe and not much higher than natural radioactivity, but soon after the Simon test in the Nevada Test Site on April 25, 1953, high levels of radioactivity were detected in Albany and Troy in New York state, where the fallout was intense and samples of tap water in Albany revealed radioactivity levels 2,630 times higher than normal.[13]

Ten years after the atomic testing had begun, populations living downwind began to experience clusters of childhood leukemia, at the time 90% fatal.[14] Many years later, in 1982, a Public Health Service radiation safety monitor who worked in Utah during the 1953 testing series, Frank Butrico, testified in a wrongful death suit filed by relatives of 24 cancer victims. Mr. Butrico testified that his instruments were "off the scales" after a particularly heavy fallout from a test nicknamed Dirty Harry, and told the court that the staff at the Nevada Test Site had told him to report only that "radiation levels were a little bit above normal but not in the range of being harmful." Later, Mr. Butrico testified that he had discovered that his reports on levels of radioactivity had been tampered with by AEC officials.

In secrecy, the AEC had initiated studies of health problems in the Japanese A-bomb survivors. The systematic gathering of data had not begun, however, until 1950, five years after the bombing, when much of the information was already irrecoverable. The data collected, secret and censored for years,[15] were an-

---

12 US Congress, House Committee on Interstate and Foreign Commerce, Subcommittee on Oversight and Investigations (1980), *Low-level radiation effects on health: hearings before the Subcommittee on Oversight and Investigations of the Committee on Interstate and Foreign Commerce, House of Representatives, 96th Congress, 1st session, April 23, May 24, and August 1, 1979, v.*

13 Rice (2015), "Downwind of the atomic state: US continental atmospheric testing, radioactive fallout, and organizational deviance, 1951–1962", *Social Science History* 39, 647–676.

14 Ball (1986), "Downdwind from the bomb", *The New York Times Magazine* Feb. 9, 33.

15 Ingram et al. (1952), *Biological effects of ionizing radiation – Sponsored by the US Atomic Energy Commission* (Declassified 3/15/13).

alyzed by the US military during the 1950s, the early years of the Cold War and a time when the US, the USSR, and the UK performed dozens of nuclear tests that released huge amounts of radiation into the atmosphere.[16] Governments insisted however that the doses of radiation received by the population from these tests were very low, negligible, and harmless. Consistently with this view, the US government announced the atomic tests and even broadcasted one on TV, and crowds in Las Vegas watched the mushroom clouds of atomic bombs exploded a hundred kilometers away.[17]

Immediately after World War II, scientists, including some who had participated in the development of the atomic bomb, started to make known the danger that nuclear weapons and radioactivity represented for humanity. Many who had participated in the Manhattan Project were seriously worried about the prospects for the world.[18] In 1946 the Emergency Committee of Atomic Scientists was founded by Albert Einstein and Leo Szilard, to warn the public of the dangers associated with the development of nuclear weapons and to promote the peaceful use of nuclear energy and world peace. Evidence that radioactivity was spreading and accumulating in the atmosphere was soon available. Radioactive carbon-14 in the atmosphere, for instance, increased by about 5% between the end of 1953 and the spring of 1957, and the increase was known to be due to atomic bomb tests.[19] In 1952 Linus Pauling, who had begun to actively criticize the development of nuclear weapons was denied a passport by the US Department of State when he was invited to speak at a scientific conference in London. He received the Nobel Prize in Chemistry in 1954, and in an statement in 1957 he estimated 10,000 people had already died or were dying of leukemia because of nuclear testing, an estimate that was supported by biologist E. B. Lewis in a paper published in *Science*.[20] Soon after, Pauling claimed that some 100,000 deaths from cancer and other diseases were to be expected from the worldwide fallout of each H-bomb tested in the atmosphere.[21] These assertions were dismissed as alarmist by governments strongly committed to the nuclear program

16 Brodie (2015), "Radiation secrecy and censorship after Hiroshima and Nagasaki", *Journal of Social History* 48(4), 842–864; Lifton & Mitchell (1995), *Hiroshima*.

17 Foner (2006), *Give me liberty! An American history*, 797–798.

18 Feynman (1998), *The meaning of it all – Thoughts of a citizen scientist*.

19 De Vries & Waterbolk (1958), "Groningen Radiocarbon Dates III", *Science* 128(3338), 1550–1556.

20 Kirsch (2004), "Harold Knapp and the geography of normal controversy: Radioiodine in the historical environment", *Osiris* 19, 167–181.

21 The first edition of Pauling's *No more war!* was published in 1958.

and attempting to reassure the public that the fallout of nuclear tests in inhabited areas represented trivial and irrelevant exposures to radioactivity.

In 1955 a paper by Gordon M. Dunning, of the Division of Biology and Medicine, AEC, titled "Protecting the public during weapons testing at the Nevada Test Site" was published in *JAMA*, the leading medical journal.[22] Following five pages of wordy technicalities and empty statements on the high scientific and medical qualifications of the personnel monitoring the potential health effects of the atomic tests, Dunning concluded that

> after five major series of nuclear weapons tests at the Nevada test site no one has incurred radiation exposures off-site that may be considered anywhere near hazardous. It is true that fall-out caused beta burns on some cows in the spring of 1952 and also some horses in 1953. The cows were 15 to 20 miles from ground zero and the horses at a lesser distance. There were no other ill-effects except for a skin damage. There have never been any reported cases of beta burns on people.

Even though the AEC already had information about the increased incidence of cancer and leukemia among Japanese survivors of the 1945 atomic bombings, neither "cancer" nor "leukemia" appeared even once in Dunning's paper, that was reprinted and widely distributed by the AEC. That Dunning was lying in the pages of *JAMA* was obvious given the fact that he had received "his battlefield baptism" in the AEC three years before, in 1952, when he deftly "deactivated" evidence showing that three civilians — postmistress Marjorie Percher and two girls, Theryl Stewart and Silva Ann Hines, all of whom died of cancer — had been exposed to dangerous doses of radiation. Dunning had also been the AEC organizer of a campaign to convince skeptical veterinarians in 1953 that unspecified causes unrelated to radiation — toxic weeds and malnutrition were mentioned but never verified — had killed 5,000 sheep that had eaten grass spiked with fresh fallout.[23]

In personnel charts of the AEC Gordon Dunning was listed as a low-level official in charge of radiation safety issues, but plenty of evidence demonstrates that he had authority to manage and suppress information about the radiation released by the testing of nuclear weapons.[24] Despite appearing often in publi-

---

22 Dunning (1955), "Protecting the public during weapons testing at the Nevada test site", *JAMA* 158(11), 900–904.
23 Udall (1994), *The Myths of August: A Personal Exploration of Our Tragic Cold War Affair with the Atom*, 226.
24 US Congress, House Committee on Interstate and Foreign Commerce, Subcommittee on Oversight and Investigations (1980), *Low-level radiation effects on health*, 297–298; Fradkin 1998, *Fallout* 187–193; Udall 1994, *The Myths*, 230–234.

cations and AEC documents as a health physicist, Dunning lacked any specific scientific background on radiation. He was a Lieutenant Colonel in the US Army, and began to work for the AEC in 1951.[25] Pulitzer Prize winner and radioactive fallout journalist researcher Philip Fradkin suggested Dunning could be an intelligence officer inside the AEC.[26] Whatever the case, he was fully knowledgeable of all the effects of the fallout, for instance that large numbers of sheep were dying and that deformed lambs were being born around the testing site.

Between May 27 and June 3, 1957, the Joint Committee on Atomic Energy of the US Congress held hearings on "The nature of radioactive fallout and its effects on man". The hearings were probably triggered by rancher complaints and statements by reputed scientists who were claiming that radioactivity from a number of different sources including atomic tests was a major hazard for human health. When Dr Charles L. Dunham, Director of the Division of Biology and Medicine of the AEC, was asked about these statements, he replied that there were differences of opinions on some issues, that other scientists had other views. He reassured the committee that after the tragic experiences in the 1910s with lethal effects of radioactivity from radium in workers painting watches, everybody had been particularly careful and he did not believe that anybody associated with the AEC program, or the Manhattan Project would have experienced any such radiation effect.[27] Another expert at the hearings was Herman J. Muller, a Nobel laureate geneticist who had discovered the mutational effects of ionizing radiation in the 1920s. In quite a different tone Muller declared that there had been

> a curious official silence concerning findings showing that the main damage to the exposed individuals themselves by small or moderate exposures to radioactive substances or X-rays consists of an insidious weakening of the body's resistance to the onset of infirmities and diseases of all kinds, expressing itself in a shortening of the length of life, and also consists in a long delayed production of certain specific disorders of which the most important are leukemia and some other malignant conditions. Still less publicized has been the increasing evidence that the amount of these effects is simply proportional to the total dose of radiation received, even when this has been given in tiny bits scattered over long periods. That is evidence for the conclusion that there is no threshold.[28]

---

25 US Congress, House Committee on Interstate and Foreign Commerce, Subcommittee on Oversight and Investigations (1980), *Low-level radiation effects on health*, 170
26 Fradkin (1998), *Fallout*, 187.
27 US Congress, Joint Committee on Atomic Energy, Special Subcommittee on Radiation (1958), *The nature of radioactive fallout and its effects on man*, 18–19.
28 US Congress, Joint Committee on Atomic Energy (1958), *The nature of radioactive fallout*, 1049.

Muller said that in his view the shortening of the length of life was extremely important, so that this together with

> the long delayed malignancies such as leukemia constitute by far the greatest damage of all the effects of radiation on the exposed individual himself. That is, of moderate and small doses. I am not speaking of the radiation sickness and death that occurs from very high exposures such as direct atomic bombing.[29]

Muller explained that in many Japanese survivors of the bomb at Hiroshima, cataracts could be observed in parts of the eye lens where cells had clearly been badly damaged, though that damage did not appear until much later after exposure when the cell divided. According to Muller this was observed in the eye lens

> because the lens is a transparent tissue. I think there is reason to believe that this happens in all the tissues of the body that contain cells that are subject to division. These tissues would, therefore, be weakened. It is true that other undamaged cells would tend to replenish the damaged places. But that replenishment or regeneration, it is to be expected, will not be complete and perfect. Therefore, there is a certain amount of damage left [...] a generalized damage all over the body [...] expressed as a weakening of resistance to disease and infirmities of all kinds, somewhat like what occurs in aging.[30]

Muller believed that more geneticists should be involved in the assessment of the dangers of radiation exposure, as others were "not likely to admit the danger from small doses." Muller complained that many physicians had refused to acknowledge the harmful effects of low-dose radiation, which "has prevented the medical profession for 30 years from duly protecting themselves, their technicians, and their patients when X-rays are used medically, and that has thereby subjected the reproductive cells of our population to very much more radiation than that from fallout".[31]

Gordon Dunning was a major figure in the 1957 hearings, in which he provided abundant technical information on radiation, and entertained the members of the subcommittee with an exercise examining in detail the radiation aspects of a hypothetical attack with four atomic bombs dropped on Washington DC. Dunning explained that in the more than 60 nuclear tests conducted by the US since 1951 at the Marshall Islands in the Pacific Ocean and in the Nevada

---

29 US Congress, Joint Committee on Atomic Energy (1958), *The nature of radioactive fallout*, 1051

30 US Congress, Joint Committee on Atomic Energy (1958), *The nature of radioactive fallout*, 1053–1055.

31 US Congress, Joint Committee on Atomic Energy (1958), *The nature of radioactive fallout*, 1062.

Test Site, the fallout on inhabitants of the Marshall Islands and Japanese fisher-
men in 1954 had been the major harmful effect off the testing areas; the only
other off-site damage had been in the US, where blast waves had caused
minor structural damage and fallout had caused skin burns on some horses
and cattle grazing within 20 miles of ground zero. About $30,000 had been
paid in claims for these damages.[32] But the maximum permissible exposures
for individuals, 50 roentgens up to age 30, Dunning noted, was much higher
than the highest fallout exposure around the Nevada Test Site which to date
had been "near Bunkerville, in 1953, where the people might have accumulated
7 to 8 roentgens of exposure".[33]

As pointed out by critics of atomic weapons many years later, both the "maximum permissible exposures" to ionizing radiation and the estimates of radiation received by people around the nuclear test sites were established in secret
by the AEC itself, and very probably with major contributions of Dunning.[34] A
method to estimate average biological doses received from fallout was developed
by Dunning himself. It required correcting a calculated incident dose for shield-
ing, for weathering and for other factors which strongly reduced the estimated
quantity of received radiation actually absorbed by the body; then, in a second
step, levels measured in different places were averaged. With this method, measurements that had indicated radioactivity levels well above the 3.9 rads considered as permissible by the AEC itself and that suggested a cumulative dose as
high as 19.6 rads during 1953 around St. George, Utah, were reduced to an estimated exposure that was not above 2.5 rads.[35] Afterwards this approach was considered as highly questionable, as average doses hide large dose amounts received in specific areas.[36]

A 20-page Summary-Analysis of the hearings of May-June 1957 was printed in
August 1957,[37] in advance of the 2200 pages of the transcripts of the hearings that
were released in 1958. The two-page "Summary of Key Points" stated that all nuclear explosions produce radioactivity though certain kinds of explosions "pro-

---

32 US Congress, Joint Committee on Atomic Energy (1958), *The nature of radioactive fallout*, 178
33 US Congress, Joint Committee on Atomic Energy (1958), *The nature of radioactive fallout*, 209.
34 Fradkin (1998), *Fallout*, 200 – 201.
35 Udall (1994), *The Myths*, 232 – 233.
36 US Congress, House Committee on Interstate and Foreign Commerce, Subcommittee on Oversight and Investigations (1980), *Low-level radiation effects on health: Hearings before the Subcommittee on Oversight and Investigations of the Committee on Interstate and Foreign Commerce,
House of Representatives, 96th Congress, 1ˢᵗ session, April 23, May 24, and August 1, 1979*, 176 – 178.
37 US Congress, Joint Committee on Atomic Energy, Special Subcommittee on Radiation (1957),
*Summary-Analysis of Hearings May 27 – 29, and June 3 – 7, 1957, The Nature of Radioactive Fallout
and Its Effects on Man.*

duce very much less radioactivity than others"; that there was general agreement that any amount of radiation increases mutations in a population, but there was a difference of opinion as to whether a very small dose of radiation would produce an increased incidence of conditions such as leukemia or bone cancer, or a decrease in life expectancy; that the consequences of further testing over the next several generations at the level of testing of the past 5 years could constitute a hazard to the world's population; and that the hearings had shown that man's exposure to fallout radiation "is and will be in general small, *for the testing already done*, compared with his exposure to other, 'normal background' sources of radiation (a fraction of 1% to 10%), and even compared with variations in 'normal background' sources"; but there were "differences of opinion on how to forecast the consequences of further testing", with the differences hardest to reconcile concerning the biological effects of radiation.

The summary was reassuring about the effects of atomic weapon tests. The fallout radiation was presented as small compared with natural background radiation, even less than 10% of it, a comforting idea that was repeated many times by the AEC, for instance in a brochure on *Fallout from nuclear tests* authored by C. L. Comar, published in 1963 and republished in 1966. This document acknowledged disagreement among scientists about the potential hazard of fallout but explained that "the extent of disagreement on this question is far less than the very extensive area of agreement". Furthermore, the "consensus of informed individuals is that the present or anticipated levels of radiation exposure from fallout due to nuclear tests (through 1962) do not constitute a hazard that warrants anxiety. There is also general agreement that fallout from nuclear testing contributes in a small way to worldwide radiation exposure". High fallout "that might result from combinations of circumstances" was to be further investigated, but scientists, private institutions, governmental agencies, and international organizations "are well aware of these matters and are actively engaged in research to reduce the uncertainties."

Reassurances from the AEC on the safety of atomic tests were contested, though, and more voices became involved in the controversies. Edward Teller and Albert Latter, advocates of the nuclear weapons and the nuclear test program insisted that for the average American, the cancer-causing radionuclides from tests amounted to a dosage of a small fraction of 1 roentgen. With tests continuing, they argued in 1958 in the pages of the popular magazine *Life*, radiation levels might increase "as much as fivefold," but even in this case it would be extremely unlikely that anyone would receive a lifetime dosage of as much as 5 roentgens, a small amount that, if it actually "does increase a person's chance of getting bone cancer or leukemia, the increase is so slight it cannot be measured." In the same magazine, Pauling disputed Teller and Latter's views as either

false or misleading. Focusing on the "average American," Pauling wrote, ob-
scured the specificity of fallout patterns, including the hotspots that, though
by no means limited to areas immediately downwind, were nevertheless dispro-
portionate located in Nevada and Utah. Pauling argued that it was not at all unlikely that lifetime doses would be over 5 roentgens, and he cited as evidence an
AEC report listing towns in Nevada and Utah where thousands of inhabitants
had already been exposed to more than 5 roentgens of fallout from a single
test series in Nevada.[38]

In the 1950s, the AEC as an organization systematically ignored the major
problem of radiation from internal isotopes absorbed from the food or inhaled.
But others didn't. Harold Knapp, a mathematician working for the Fallout
Branch of the AEC Division of Biology and Medicine, produced estimates of io-
dine-131 (I-131) in cow milk and in human thyroid in places around the Nevada
Test Site that strongly conflicted with AEC estimates produced by Dunning. Dunning tried to stop the publication of Knapp's estimates, and Knapp was dismissed from the AEC, but he forced the AEC to publish his report and also published his findings in *Nature*.[39] In 1979 Knapp testified at congressional hearings
on effects of low-dose radiation, and described in straightforward terms how radiation from the fallout could perfectly explain the 1953 deaths of several thousand sheep in Nevada and Utah.[40] Knapp estimated that the thyroid dose to a
one-year-old child in Fruitland, Utah, from a nuclear test in June 1962, could
have been more than 130 times the annual radiation protection guidelines established at the time. He also estimated I-131 in fallout in the 1950s, and extrapolating I-131 levels from existing measurements, calculated the uptake of I-131 in cow
milk, arriving to the conclusion that from just one 1953 test, infants who had
been living in a radiation hotspot, St. George, Utah, might well have received
I-131 doses anywhere from 150 to 750 times what at the time was considered
an annual permissible dose.

Despite the secrecy and PR initiatives of the AEC, outrage on nuclear tests
grew in the late 1950s and early 1960s, fueled by reports of substantial doses
of radioactivity from the tests in New Mexico and Nevada reaching the East
coast and lawsuits from ranchers and residents in Nevada, Utah and Minneso-

38 Kirsch (2004), "Harold Knapp and the geography of normal controversy: Radioiodine in the
historical environment", *Osiris* 19, 167–181.
39 Knapp (1964), "Iodine-131 in fresh milk and human thyroids following a single deposition of
nuclear test fall-out", *Nature* 202(4932), 534–537.
40 US Congress, Joint Committee on Atomic Energy (1958), *The nature of radioactive fallout*,
299–311.

ta.[41] All this undoubtedly contributed to the signing of the 1963 Partial Test Ban Treaty, which banned all nuclear tests above ground, in the atmosphere, underwater and in outer space. Nuclear weapon testing underground, though, not only continued but increased in the following years. A total of 928 nuclear tests have been conducted at the Nevada Test Site to date. Worldwide, over 2,000 nuclear tests have been conducted by eight nations (Table 7.1) with some 500 of these atomic tests conducted in the atmosphere, thus launching huge quantities of radioactivity that passed from the air to the ground and the trophic chains.

Tab. 7.1: Nuclear tests conducted to date worldwide. The total is over 2,000 tests including some 500 tests in the atmosphere

Country	Period	Total	Atmospheric	Location
USA	1945–1992	1054	216[a]	New Mexico, Japan,[b] Pacific Ocean Nevada Test Site
USSR	1949–1990	715[c]	219[a]	USSR territory[d]
United Kingdom	1952–1991	45?	45?	Australia, Pacific Ocean, Nevada[e]
France	1960–1996	210	50	Algeria and Polynesia
China	1964–1996	45	23	All in Xinjiang, one in Inner Mongolia
India	1974, 1998	6?	0	Pokhran, Rajahkstan, India
Pakistan	1983?-1998	6?	0	Ras Koh, Pakistan
North Korea	2006–2017	6	0	Punggye-ri Test Site, North Korea
South Africa	1979	1?	1	Indian Ocean

[a] This number includes some underwater and space tests.
[b] This refers to the bombs on Hiroshima and Nagasaki, assuming them as "tests."
[c] This includes a total of 969 devices, as some tests were "salvo tests" in which several devices were exploded simultaneously.
[d] Most tests were conducted in present-day Kazakhstan, some in the Artic Ocean (Novyaa Zemlya) and present-day independent republics of Uzbekistan, Ukraine, and Turkmenistan.
[e] The total of 45 tests includes 12 in Australian territory, 9 in the Line Islands of the central Pacific and 24 in the US as part of joint test series. Often excluded from British totals are the 31 safety tests of Operation Vixen in Maralinga, Australia.
Source: Author's elaboration from data in multiple sources.

The end of atmospheric tests in Nevada did not end criticisms of the AEC during the 1960s. AEC 's regulations were considered insufficiently rigorous in areas re-

---

41 Blitz (2016), "When Kodak accidentally discovered A-bomb testing", *Popular Mechanics* June 20; Honicker (1987), *Premeditated deceit: The Atomic Energy Commission against Joseph August Sauter.*

lated to radiation effects, including radiation protection standards, nuclear reactor safety, plant siting, and environmental protection. In 1974 the US Congress abolished the AEC by the Energy Reorganization Act of 1974, which assigned its functions to two new agencies: the Energy Research and Development Administration and the Nuclear Regulatory Commission.

According to the historian Eric Foner, the Cold War encouraged a culture of secrecy and dishonesty. Not until decades later was it revealed that during the 1950s and 1960s both the Soviet and American governments conducted experiments in which unwitting soldiers were exposed to chemical, biological, and nuclear weapons. American nuclear tests, conducted on Pacific islands and in Nevada, exposed the population at large to radiation that caused cancer and birth defects.[42]

For Stewart Lee Udall, who served three terms as a congressman from Arizona and then as Secretary of the Interior under presidents Kennedy and Johnson, what the AEC did in the 1950s was a classic cover-up that

> evolved into the most long-lived program of public deception in US history. Each lie generated additional misconduct and additional lies, and any search for evidence concerning the decisions that initiated the cover-up hit a blank wall. Cover-ups invariably engender illusions that warp the judgment of those who participate in them. When AEC officials embraced the idea that their efforts would be discredited and disrupted if they admitted radiation dangers, they entered a moral wasteland. Decision-making was perverted; twisted reasoning fostered a conviction that it was more important to protect the tests than to protect civilians. Any cover-up must be enforced by designated agents, and one man emerged in 1953 as the quarterback of the AEC's damage control. His name was Gordon Dunning.[43]

Until the 1980s when Gorbachev's *glasnost* was implemented, an utter secrecy on the details of the development of nuclear weapons, nuclear tests and nuclear energy prevailed in the Soviet Union, where large releases of radioactivity because of tests, accidents, and the production of nuclear fuel occurred long before Chernobyl and were hidden for decades.[44] However, in many ways the Chernobyl disaster motivated an alignment of the interests of the governments of the East and the West in the defense of the "safety" of atomic power. The evolution of knowledge about the consequences of the Chernobyl disaster since the 1990s — which

---

42 Foner (2006), *Give me liberty!*, 797.
43 Udall (1994), *The Myths*, 234.
44 Simons (1993), "Soviet atom test used thousands as guinea pigs, archives show", *The New York Times*, Nov. 7, 1, 20; Brown (2013), *Plutopia: Nuclear families, atomic cities, and the great Soviet and American plutonium disasters*; Mahaffey (2014), *Atomic accidents: A history of nuclear meltdowns and disasters: From the Ozark mountains to Fukushima*.

will be examined in the following chapters — shows many similarities with how the initial reports and assessments by the AEC and the US atomic *establishment* were progressively discredited over time leading eventually to the disappearance of the AEC.

During the Clinton presidency a commission was organized to evaluate the effects of radiation on humans. The activities and report of that commission led to a public apology by the President and indemnification payments. Among the victims of the experiments with radiation that were performed on human beings were the soldiers who were exposed to acute radiation in areas close to nuclear tests in Nevada.[45]

---

45 Faden (1996), " The Advisory Committee on Human Radiation Experiments: Reflections on a Presidential Commission", *The Hastings Center Report* 26(5), 5–10; in Youtube there are multiples videos of impressive footage from the atomic tests in Nevada (e. g., www.youtube.com/watch?v=53EPfK56y48; www.youtube.com/watch?v=-8pIpB2lf-A).

Chapter 8
Effects of low-dose radiation — The LNT model — Hormesis

Knowledge about the relation between the dose of something and the effect of that exposure on some specific outcome begins with observations. From the analysis of these observations a model describing the relation between levels of the exposure and their effects is derived. Further observations validate that model, or when new observations do not fit the predictions of the model, the analyst is forced to modify the model, or discard it in full and start from scratch trying to build a new model. In biomedical sciences and epidemiology, linearity is the simplest dose-effect model and often fits the data very well. The effect of an exposure on a risk is linear when the risk is proportional to the exposure, so that, for instance, halving the exposure will halve the risk. Thus, as shown in Fig. 8.1, observations of the risk of cancer as a function of smoking fit a linear model quite well, so that if a given exposure to cigarette smoke generates an x cancer risk, then half the exposure will generate an $x/2$ risk.[1] There is no exposure level below which risk is zero, so this model is referred to as a linear no-threshold or LNT model.

Let's now assume that we have observations for four levels of exposure to a given physical or chemical agent and the corresponding levels of risk of developing a given outcome. The four measurements for exposures are 16, 21, 32, and 42, and the respective measured risks are 2.0, 2.6, 3.5, and 5.0 (no matter the units). Figs. 8.2, 8.3 and 8.4, show these four observations as dots. Now, considering such observations, what would be the risk for a low-dose exposure of say 5 units? To answer that question, we first need a model of the risk as a function of the exposure. Once a particular model is assumed, we then use the model to extrapolate what the outcome would be for an exposure of 5 units (a level of exposure below the lowest level that we actually observed). Since our four hypothetical observations are reasonably placed on a straight line, we can assume the risk is a linear function, directly proportional to the exposure, in which case the exposure at a dose of 5 implies a risk of 0.74, as shown in Fig. 8.2. For a polynomial quadratic model, as in Fig. 8.3, which has a slightly better fit than the linear (as shown by a higher R^2) the estimated risk is higher, 1.53. Finally for the logarithmic model shown in Fig. 8.4, the expected risk for 5 units of exposure is negative, -1.61, which means that at such level, the exposure would be protec-

---

1 Bonita et al. (2008), *Basic epidemiology.*

https://doi.org/10.1515/9783110761788-012

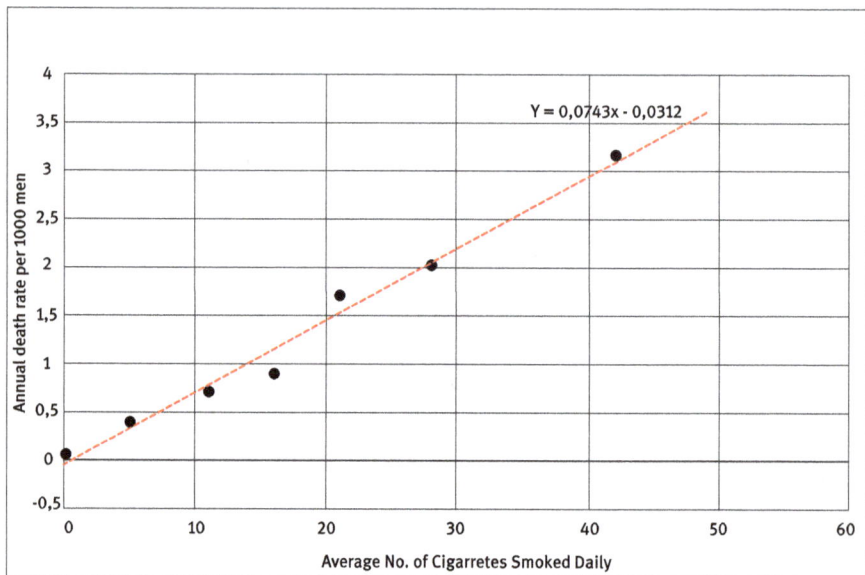

Fig. 8.1: Death rate from lung cancer, standardized for age, among men smoking different daily numbers of cigarettes at the start of the inquiry. Data taken from a figure in Doll & Hill (1950).

tive of the risk; there would be also a threshold level, because in that model the risk is null or negative for exposures of 8.55 or lower. Of course, more models are possible, the three presented here are just the simplest ones, and simplicity, is often referred to as the application of Occam's razor and generally considered as a desirable characteristic of scientific theories.

The linear no-threshold (LNT) model for effects of radiation

Scientists dealing with the estimation of the potential effects of ionizing radiation at low doses have had to deal with theoretical problems related to the identification of the right model. This became especially pressing after the emergence of sources of radiation that exposed many people to low doses. Before World War II the main use of ionizing radiation was the medical diagnostic or treatment procedures of physicians and dentists who were confidently exposing many people to low or not so low doses of X-rays. However, the early development of radiological techniques had been plagued by health problems. Around 1900 Thomas Edison was developing a fluoroscope that appeared to be almost ready for

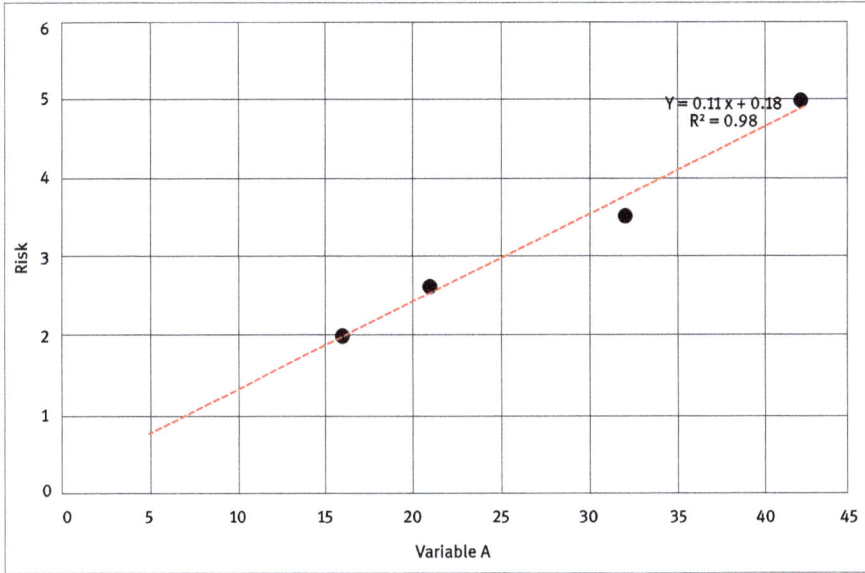

Fig. 8.2: Risk as a linear function.

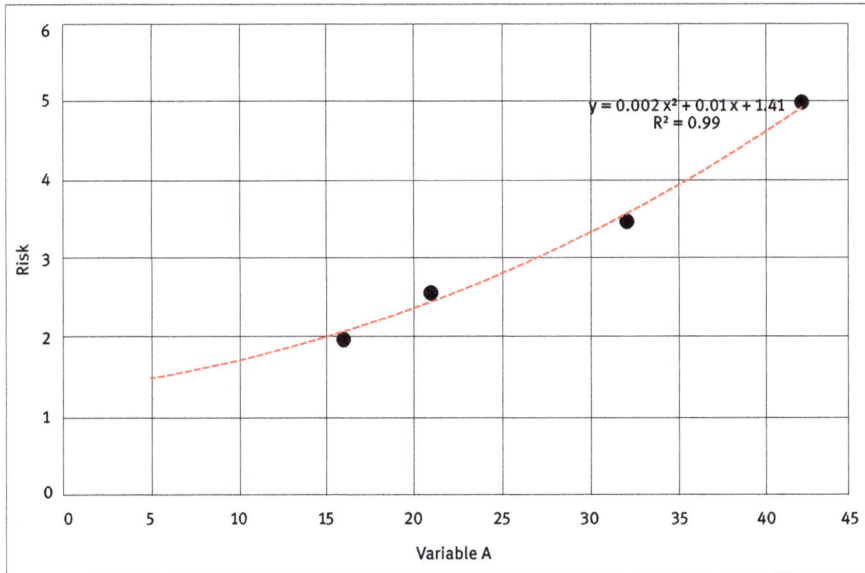

Fig. 8.3: Risk as a polinomial function.

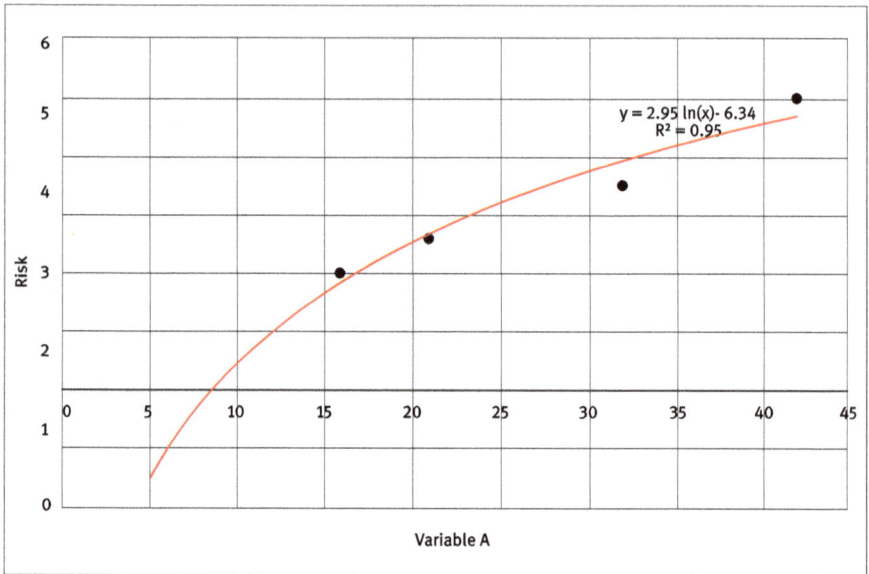

Fig. 8.4: Risk as a logarithmic function.

commercialization when he had to abandon his research on this device because of the health hazards of radiation exposure. He damaged an eye in testing his devices and Clarence Dally, one Edison's technician who was repeatedly exposed, suffered radiation poisoning, and later died of cancer.[2] Maria Salomea Skłodowska, usually known as Madame Curie, died in 1934, aged 66, of aplastic anemia attributed to her exposure to radiation during her scientific research and her radiological work during World War I. The death of her daughter Irène (1897–1956) and her daughter's husband Frédéric Joliot (1900–1958) is today believed to have been also caused by radioactivity.[3] In the early decades of the 20th century, though, radioactive sources, radium especially, were present in multiple everyday products, including radioactive creams for skin rejuvenation, as well as radioactive elixirs that were marketed to clean the body of toxins and disease. Mineral waters for drinking were promoted as being radioactive, which at the time was considered a major advantage.

---

2 Radiopaedia, "Thomas Edison".
3 Wikipedia, "Pierre Curie", Baldwin & Grantham (2015), "Radiation hormesis: Historical and current perspectives", *Journal of Nuclear Medicine Technology* 43(4), 242–246.

The use of radium to paint luminous dials in clocks and measurement in-struments mostly manufactured for the military during the First World War caused the first case of occupational exposure to radioactivity, with hundreds of osteosarcomas and other cancers detected in the 1920s in the workers, mostly woman, exposed to radium.[4] Then came World War II, with the A-bombs on Hir-oshima and Nagasaki that exposed many tens of thousands to radioactive fall-out. In the following years sources of exposure to ionizing radiation multiplied, including the medical exposure of doctors and patients, the occupational expo-sure of miners and workers involved in the extraction and processing of radio-active materials, and the exposure resulting from the fallout of nuclear tests that began to be conducted in the late 1940s at a rate of several per year, and sometimes per month, by both the United States and the USSR. Most of these sources were allegedly producing low-dose exposure to ionizing radiation, but the population exposed was large, millions of people; in fact, everyone on Earth.

Ever since the studies by Herman Muller in the 1920s on the mutagenic prop-erties of ionizing radiation, there was no theoretical reason to believe that doses of radiation below some level would be absolutely safe. Despite this, many doc-tors and dentists had been using X-rays since the 1910s and two decades later they were still confident that exposures to doses sufficiently low would be harm-less.

Since the 1950s or even earlier, the LNT model was considered to be the sim-plest and most appropriate way to describe the relation between radiation re-ceived and risk of mutation in general or malignancy in particular since the 1950s, or even earlier.[5] By 1954, according to A. H. Sturtevant, who was at the time president of the Pacific Division of the American Association for the Ad-vancement of Science, it was "widely confirmed" that radiogenic mutations in reproductive cells appeared at a frequency proportional to the dosage of radia-tion; there was almost certainly no threshold value below which radiation was insignificant for that purpose; and the genetic effects of radiation were cumula-tive and permanent. As Sturtevant put it, these observations were "so widely confirmed that we may confidently assert that they apply to all higher organisms including man".[6] However, as Herman Muller explained in the congressional

---

4 Polednak (1978), "Bone cancer among female radium dial workers. Latency periods and inci-dence rates by time after exposure", *Journal of the National Cancer Institute* 60(1), 77–82.
5 Russell et al. (1958), "Radiation dose rate and mutation frequency", *Science* 128(3338), 1546–1550; US Congress, Joint Committee on Atomic Energy, Special Subcommittee on Radiation 1958, *The nature of radioactive fallout and its effects on man*, 1049–1085.
6 Kirsch (2004), "Harold Knapp and the geography of normal controversy: Radioiodine in the historical environment", *Osiris* 19, 167–181.

hearings of 1957 on atomic energy and radiation, although geneticists were in agreement on the validity of the LNT model, not all scientists were in agreement.[7] The divisive part was mostly the NT part of the LNT, i.e, the assumption that there was no-threshold. Note that in theory the straight line representing a linear model could intersect the horizontal axis at a positive value in which case there would be a threshold and effects would be zero or negative (that is, beneficial, with a reduction in risk), at levels of exposure below the threshold.

Scientific committees appointed by governments in the 1950s to set standards for radiation were strongly biased toward the idea that low-level doses were harmless, as at the time for most in the medical profession a low level of exposure to ionizing radiation in radiography or fluoroscopy was considered innocuous. Many radiation experts were working for governments in the development and construction of atomic weapons; others worked for private companies in developing commercial applications of ionizing radiation or atomic energy. These scientists, many of whom had a sincere interest in harnessing and finding peaceful applications of this newly discovered and for many at the time "marvelous" form of energy had both professional and financial interests in being blind to the effects of low-dose radiation. For industries using nuclear technologies that generated radiation and for governments performing nuclear tests that disseminated radioactive fallout there was an overarching interest to convince the public that radiation — either from medical or dental practices or from any other source — had no risk. On TV, and in radio and newspapers, stories suggested that soon each household would have an atomic reactor which would provide for electricity, heating and refrigeration and all the energy requirements of the modern family; nuclear energy would move airplanes, ships and cars, and would be usable for the excavation of mines and construction of channels.[8] "Low-dose radiotherapy" was used to treat almost anything, including all kind of inflammatory processes, acne, fungi in the scalp (*tinea capitis*), and menstrual disorders. X-rays fluoroscopy for diagnostic purposes was widespread in medical practice for all kind of patients. It was more and more common to X-ray pregnant women to determine the position of their babies and X-ray fluoroscopes were used commercially to fit shoes to children and adults.[9]

---

7 US Congress, Joint Committee on Atomic Energy, Special Subcommittee on Radiation (1958), *The nature of radioactive fallout and its effects on man*, 1958, 1049–1062.

8 Anonymous (1955), "Calefacción y refrigeración por medio de un pequeño reactor nuclear", *El Telegrama del Rif* (Melilla, Spain), 3 de junio, 1; Udall (1994), *The myths of August*, 136–141, 255.

9 Wikipedia, "Shoe-fitting fluoroscope", Healio Hematology-Oncology, "The shoe fitting fluoroscope, a little-known application of the X ray".

(I can't resist intruding here with two episodes from my own experience related to the reckless use of radiation for medical purposes which was so common five decades ago and that to some extent still exists. I was 5 years old, living in Granada, Spain. Because a friend of my father was a reputed radiologist, I had "the privilege" of being examined several times with X-ray fluoroscopy together with other children, we all watched the "skeletons" with amusement. Sixteen or seventeen years later a medical student, I developed a sore throat and hoarse voice that lasted many weeks. The ENT specialist told me I had a chronic laryngitis. He prescribed vitamins but told me this could be very well treated with radiotherapy, though this was not covered by the medical school insurance I had — so I would have to pay out of pocket, which I did not accept. At the time I was smoking two packs a day which is an obvious reason for having a chronic laryngitis, but the ENT doctor said nothing about smoking, instead he suggested "radiotherapy" that fortunately I did not accept.)

With the passage of time these kinds of "low-dose" medical or non-medical uses of radiation were acknowledged as carcinogenic. The quotation marks around "low dose" are appropriate because fluoroscopy usually represents a dose equivalent to hundreds of X-ray radiographs. A British doctor, Alice Mary Stewart, had an important role in the recognition of the effects of low-dose radiation. Incidence of leukemia in children was rising in the 1950s and some suggested that this could be related to environmental factors. Dr. Stewart was surprised when, after questioning many mothers, she found that the children of mothers who had had X-rays were almost twice as likely as other children to develop cancer. Doctors and the nuclear industry were outraged by the publication of this finding, it could not be true that receiving such a low dose of radiation was harmful. Dr. Stewart had difficulties obtaining funding for other studies but in subsequent years other scientists replicated her findings and prenatal X-rays were recognized as harmful and abandoned.[10] Dr Stewart's finding was consistent with the view that there is no threshold for the mutational effect of radiation. As early as 1957 the Surgeon General of the US strongly recommended avoiding radiography and fluoroscopy in screening programs of tuberculosis, and additional recommendations limiting the use of these applications of radiation were passed by the FDA as recently as 2009.[11]

In a book published in 1992 John Gofman estimated that about three quarters of all breast cancers in the US are caused by medical X-rays. According to

10 Greene (2017), *The woman who knew too much: Alice Stewart and the secrets of radiation*; Richmond (2002), "Alice Mary Stewart", *BMJ* 325(7355), 106.
11 FDA, "Fluoroscopy", accessed March 2020.

Gofman, professor of molecular and cell biology at Berkeley, and expert in radio-active substances and their biological effects on living beings, information in government documents declassified in the 1990s revealed that "powerful seg-ments of the US Government were actively engaged — starting soon after Hirosh-ima and Nagasaki — in suppressing information which might cause the public to worry about radiation." This included radiation from bomb-testing fallout, from certain aspects of military service, from working in or living near certain defense industries, or from working in uranium mines. Under the circumstances prevail-ing in the 1950s, said Gofman, "it was probably not a favorable time to start teaching the public to worry about radiation from shoe-fitters".[12]

Of course, disagreements regarding the innocuous or potentially harmful character of low doses of radiation continued in the scientific field in the 1960s, the 1970s and the 1980s;[13] and indeed they persist today. The belief that low doses were innocuous or at least created a very low risk continued to be strongly held by many, and was implicit in the standards for radiation safety set in the US by the Federal Radiation Council with advice from the AEC during the 1950s and 1960s. However, "permissible dose" limits were revised downward repeatedly in 1951, 1955, 1957, and 1960.[14] Genetic studies with plants and ani-mals had showed that the number of mutations was proportional to the radiation dose, even at very low levels of radiation, and criticisms were leveled against the idea that there was a threshold below which radiation is safe, and the idea that the risk depends on the rate of application of the mutagenic agent. In 1946 Her-mann Muller had received a Nobel Prize for his work on the mutagenic effect of radiation. He had demonstrated that radiation may cause genetic mutation and suggested mutation as a cause of cancer. In his Nobel Lecture he asserted that mutation frequency is "directly and simply proportional to the dose of irradia-tion applied" (i.e., linear) and that there is "no threshold dose",[15] a view that at the time was very common among biologists. By 1956 the model of linear no-threshold (LNT) mutagenic effects of radiation had become settled genetic science as proved by its adoption by a National Academy of Sciences (NAS) panel, the genetics panel of the so-called NAS Biological Effects of Atomic Radi-

---

12 Gofman (1996), *Preventing breast cancer — The story of a major, proven, preventable cause of this disease*, chapter 27.
13 Ad hoc Working Group, US Department of Health & Human Services, Public Health Service, NIH (1985), *Report of the NIH ad hoc working group to develop radioepidemiological tables*.
14 Kirsch (2004), Harold Knapp.
15 Wikipedia, "Linear no threshold model".

ation (BEAR) Committee.[16] The committee agreed on the essence of the LNT theory, particularly that radiations cause mutations; that practically all radiation-induced mutations which are detectable are harmful; that any radiation even of small dose, can induce mutations; that mutations can arise from natural causes; that to "the best of our present knowledge, if we increase the radiation by X%, the gene mutations caused by radiation will also be increased by X%"; and that from the point of view of genetic damage, what counts is not the rate at which radiation is given, but the total accumulated dose to the reproductive cells. This general understanding was aligned with the theory that ionizing radiation damages certain molecules in cells in a stochastic fashion and with the experimental data available at the time. Linus Pauling echoed that theoretical and empirical knowledge in 1958 when he wrote that in terms of ability to produce genetic defects, it makes no difference whether the gonads are exposed to a single large dose of radiation or to many very small ones spread over a long period of time, as the number of mutations depends only on total exposure.[17]

A study published in 1962 on the leukemia experience of the Japanese survivors of atomic bombing considered it demonstrated "beyond reasonable doubt the leukaemogenic effect on man of ionizing radiation," with increased risk of leukemia after doses as low as 100 rads. Leukemia incidence was perhaps "linearly related to the radiation dose" above this level but data were too limited to evaluate the risk represented by doses at the lower levels of radiation, where a threshold dose for leukemia induction might exist.[18]

Overall evidence on the biological effects of radiation accumulated and in the 1970s there was not only experimental data showing ionizing radiation as a potent carcinogenic agent but wide epidemiological knowledge about how most cancers can be produced by radiation and how multiple types of cancer are induced through mutations in cells. Known occupational examples were leukemias and other malignancy from X-ray exposure in radiologists, lung cancer from internal alpha radiation in uranium miners and other workers in mining, osteogenic sarcomas in luminous dial painters, and lymphomas in uranium workers.[19]

---

16 Beyea (2017), "Lessons to be learned from a contentious challenge to mainstream radiobiological science", *Environmental Research* 154, 362–379.

17 Pauling (1983), *No more war!*, 68.

18 Tomonaga (1962), "Leukaemia in Nagasaki atomic bomb survivors from 1945 through 1959", *Bulletin of the World Health Organization* 26(5), 619–631.

19 Archer (1977), "Occupational exposure to radiation as a cancer hazard", *Cancer* 34(4), 1802–1806.

In the US the progressive development of agreed knowledge about the biological effects of radioactivity was marked by the publication of reports of committees of the National Academy of Sciences (NAS). After the 1956 NAS report on *Biological Effects of Atomic Radiation,* sometimes called BEAR I, a series of seven reports from the National Research Council (NRC) were prepared "to advise the US government on the relationship between exposure to ionizing radiation and human health".[20] This series on biological effects of ionizing radiation started with BEIR I, published in 1972. The most recent report is BEIR VII, which was published in two phases, in 1998 and 2006.

As these reports were developed, new problems and controversies appeared. Thus, the NAS committee that met in 1960 (BEAR-II) considered that the estimation of radiation hazards for humans was more difficult than it had appeared to be in 1955.[21] Since that time there had been observations that in some specific cells fewer mutations were produced by chronic irradiation than by acute irradiation when the total dose was the same. Thus, the assumed constancy of the total genetic effect irrespective of dose rate, for which there seemed to be good evidence, had turned out not to be applicable to specific cells such as spermatogonia and oocytes which are most important as far as human hazards are concerned. Showing exquisite attention to detail in considering scientific disagreements, the BEAR-II Subcommittee reported as follows:

> Prediction requires evaluation of the possibility that there is a threshold dose below which there is no probability of inducing leukemia, a concept which implies a factor of safety that would be most reassuring to those who are exposed to radiation in excess of the natural background as well as to those who must make policy decisions. Some members of the Subcommittee believe, on the basis of analogy to radium data and chemical poisons, that there must be a threshold; however, no member of the Subcommittee feels that he can estimate the size of the threshold or, for that matter, even prove its existence. Accordingly, the Subcommittee believes it is prudent to assume that there is no threshold.[22]

Considering the Japanese data on the relationship of a single dose of radiation (that of the atomic bomb) with the incidence of leukemia, the Subcommittee asserted that evidence was sufficient to predict the risk of leukemia with doses over 50 to 100 rads. Above this range, the incidence increased with dose in an approximately linear manner. But in the Japanese exposed to doses believed to be less

---

20 National Research Council (2006), *Risks from Exposure to Low Levels of Ionizing Radiation: BEIR VII Phase 2, vii.*
21 NAS-NRC, National Academy of Sciences, National Research Council (1960), *The Biological Effects of Atomic Radiation (BEAR-II) – Summary Report,* 3.
22 NAS-NRC (1960), *BEAR Summary Report,* 34.

than 50 – 100 rads, the occurrence of leukemia since 1945 was not significantly greater than in the general population. Thus, the Subcommittee was not willing to accept the assumptions of E. B. Lewis and others that there would be a continued constant incidence of leukemia per rad exposure for the duration of life and that the incidence would be identical for acute and chronic exposure, i.e., that the incidence would not depend on the dose rate.[23]

The BEAR-II subcommittee of the US NAS was thus facing an important complication in the evaluation of the biological effects of atomic radiation, to know, whether the risk depends or not on the rate or speed with which the exposure occurs, a rate which often is not easy to ascertain. If the exposure to a total of 12 units of radiation during a year generates significantly less risk of cancer 20 years later than an identical exposure to 12 units of radiation in a single exposure, say during an hour, then the risk is dependent on the dose rate. In that case, the reduction in risk is given by a dose-rate effectiveness factor (DREF). A DREF of 10 for comparing an annual dose to an acute hourly dose implies that exposure to 12 units of radiation during a year would generate only one tenth of the risk of cancer generated by an acute exposure of 12 units in an hour. Overall, the BEAR and BEIR reports, accepted the LNT model as the primary way to evaluate the health effects of low dose radiation, and according to basic tenets of radiobiology, the harm produced by radiation was thought to be dependent on the total dose. However, the introduction of DREFs was a departure of this general approach and revealed underlying difficulties.

In 1979, when the BEIR III report was being prepared, controversy arose. The models relating ionizing radiation to health effects that had been developed from data on acute exposures were increasingly believed by some to be problematic for applications to continuous low dose-rate exposures and some members of the committee considered that low-level radiation was not at all as risky as a LNT model would indicate. To accommodate some empirical observations a DREF had been introduced into the assessment of radiation effects in the past. The inclusion of this DREF would allow the effect of a total dose of radiation to be modified by the rate at which that radiation was received. In the BEIR III report DREF values substantially above 1 were proposed for some low dose exposures, indicating that the health effects would be significantly dependent on the rate at which radiation was received. The controversy around these issues delayed the publication of BEIR III to 1980.[24]

---

23 NAS-NRC (1960), *BEAR Summary Report*, 35.
24 Fabrikant (1981), "The BEIR-III Report: Origin of the controversy", *American Journal of Roentgenology* 136, 209 – 214.

In 1983 an *ad hoc* Working Group of the NIH prepared radio-epidemiological tables stating probabilities of causation for different cancers at varying levels of radiation. The resulting report stated that for acute leukemias, chronic granulo-cytic leukemia, and female breast cancer the association with ionizing radiation "is so strong as to appear certain" but it also noted that there was "fairly strong evidence that ionizing radiation does not cause chronic lymphatic leukemia".[25] For carcinogenesis, in general, and radiation carcinogenesis in particular, the re-port stated strong reasons for questioning the assumption that the dose-response relationship had a threshold and concluded that the notion of a threshold for ra-diation carcinogenesis was not tenable for purposes of risk assessment. A linear-quadratic model was used to compute radioepidemiological probabilities for leu-kemia, a model predicting "that small doses of radiation have a lesser effect per rad than do higher doses." Judging that radiobiological reasons in favor of this model were solid, the Working Group applied it to all cancer types except carci-noma of the breast and thyroid, in which a simple linear model was used. With respect to dose fractioning of low-linear-energy transfer (LET) radiation (such as β and γ radiation), the Working Group followed the prevailing recommendations of UNSCEAR, the National Council of Radiation Protection and Measurement and BEIR-III in using DREF values spaning a wide range, from 2 to 10.

In 1990 the BEIR V Report stated once again that the excess risk of non-leu-kemia cancer mortality derived from observations of Japanese survivors exposed only once to radiation (that of the A-bombs of Hiroshima and Nagasaki) fit a LNT model quite well. However, "departures from a linear model at low doses [...] could either increase or decrease the risk per unit dose".[26] Actually, the depar-ture suggested in the report was downward,[27] as it was noted that for low-LET radiation, the distribution of the same dose "over weeks or months (...) is expect-ed to reduce the life time risk appreciably, possibly by a factor 2 or more".[28] In-deed, DREF values proposed for low-LET radiation once again ranged from 2 to 10 and, for instance, the DREF for models predicting effects on life shortening had a single best estimate of 4.[29]

25 *Ad hoc* Working Group, US Department of Health & Human Services, Public Health Service, NIH 1985, *Report of the NIH ad hoc working group to develop radioepidemiological tables*, 16.
26 National Research Council (1990), *Health effects of exposure to low levels of ionizing radia-tion: BEIR V*.
27 Nussbaum & Kohnlein (1994), "Inconsistencies and open questions regarding low-dose health effects of ionizing radiation", *Environmental Health Perspectives* 102(8), 656–667.
28 National Research Council (1990), *Health Effects of Exposure to Low Levels of Ionizing Radi-ation: BEIR V*, 6.
29 National Research Council (1990), *Health Effects of Exposure*, Table 1–4.

In the 1990s the evaluation of the cancer risk from ionizing radiation underwent significant revisions, as new data became available on carcinogenic effects.[30] Not only were the individual dose estimates received by Japanese survivors of atomic bombs revised upward, but now that the follow-up period had been extended to 1985, a considerable increase in cancer deaths among the low-dose subcohorts of these Japanese subjects was documented, showing longer than expected latencies for malignant diseases. The higher estimates of the cancer risk from low-dose radiation were also supported by investigations of the carcinogenic effects of ionizing radiation in individuals undergoing fluoroscopy, women subjected to mammography in mass screening for breast cancer, patients irradiated medically, and workers exposed to radiation in various occupations.[31]

The 2006 BEIR VII Report was the next statement on the health effects of low-dose radiation.[32] DREFs were discussed in the body of the report and a new concept of DDREF, "dose and dose-rate effectiveness factor," was introduced. However, the Report-In-Brief stated that research on health effects of radiation did not support the hypothesis that low doses of radiation were more harmful than a LNT model would suggest, but also did not support the hypotheses that risks were smaller than predicted by the LNT model, or were inexistent, or that low doses of radiation were protective, as suggested by the hormesis notion.[33] Surprisingly, despite being published 30 years after Chernobyl, the term "Chernobyl" which appears abundantly in the body of the 406-page report, does not appear a single time in the four pages of the Report-In-Brief. In a box reporting the new epidemiologic information used in BEIR VII models and in other sections of the Report-In-Brief it was emphasized that studies on Hiroshima and Nagasaki survivors constituted the main source of knowledge for the effects of low-dose radiation, Chernobyl was not even mentioned. Apparently, there was a tendency to avoid mentioning the Chernobyl experience. This was also illustrated by a major paper published in 2003 in the *Proceedings of the National Academy of Sciences* assessing what was already known about how low-

---

30 Fabrikant (1991), "The carcinogenic risks of low-LET and high-LET ionizing radiations", *Journal of Radiation Research* 32(2), 143–164; Nussbaum & Kohnlein (1994), "Inconsistencies and open questions".

31 Fabrikant (1991), "The carcinogenic risks of low-LET and high-LET ionizing radiations"; Nussbaum & Kohnlein (1994), "Inconsistencies and open questions".

32 National Research Council (2006), *Health risks from exposure to low levels of ionizing radiation: BEIR VII Phase 2*.

33 National Research Council, "BEIR VII: Health risks from exposure to low levels of ionizing radiation — Report in brief", accessed June 2020.

dose radiation causes cancer.[34] In this paper the name of Chernobyl was cited only once in a table in which the dose of 14 mSv was given as total dose over a 70-year period to 0.5 million individuals in rural Ukraine in the vicinity of the Chernobyl accident, compared with 3 mSv dose for a single screening mammogram (breast dose), 25 mSv for a pediatric CT scan (stomach dose from abdominal scan) or a mean total exposure of 200 mSv for the participants in the Life-Span Study of the Japanese A-bomb survivors. For Brenner et al. it was impossible at the time to be sure of the appropriate dose-response relation to use for estimating cancer risk at very low doses:

> Mechanistic arguments exist for suggesting that a linear extrapolation of risks to very low doses is appropriate, but testing such arguments at very low doses is not easy. However, the alternate models (...), although applicable for some endpoints, are less credible than the linear model as a generic descriptor of radiation carcinogenesis at low doses and low dose rates (...). In summary, given our current state of knowledge, the most reasonable assumption is that the cancer risks from low doses of X- or gamma-rays decrease linearly with decreasing dose. In light of the evidence for downwardly curving dose responses (...), this linear assumption is not necessarily the most conservative approach (...) and it is likely that it will result in an underestimate of some radiation risks and an overestimate of others.

In the 1970s those favorable to the threshold model which would imply no risk for radiation doses below some level could argue that 20 years after Hiroshima the only health effects of low-dose ionizing radiation on survivors were thyroid cancer and leukemia.[35] The view of the ICRP and UNSCEAR at the time was that effects of low-dose radiation on the cancer risk of A-bomb survivors should be indistinguishable from the background cancer risk of the Japanese population. As it will be discussed in subsequent chapters of this book, studies of the long-term lagged effects of exposure to radiation in A-bomb survivors in Japan and in the populations exposed to Chernobyl fallout that have been published in the present century have questioned to an important extent the view that the only harmful effects of low-dose ionizing radiation on survivors were thyroid cancer and leukemia. But significant scientific disagreement around this remains. For example, there have been recent criticisms against the use of the LNT model as a valid tool to evaluate the risks from low-dose radiation by authors who consider it an obsolete tool and attack it as lacking any connection

---

34 Brenner et al. (2003), "Cancer risks attributable to low doses of ionizing radiation: Assessing what we really know", *PNAS* 100(24), 137–61.
35 Baverstock & Williams (2006), "The Chernobyl accident 20 years on — An assessment of the health consequences and the international response", *Environmental Health Perspectives* 114, 1312–1317.

with radiobiological evidence.[36] Authors who question the LNT model are often in favor of the notion of hormesis.[37] For example:

> In contrast to the LNT paradigm's insistence that all radiation is harmful and the harm is cumulative, no matter how low the dose or dose rate, the school of radiation science that is based in evolutionary biology and recognizes the very widespread phenomenon of hormesis holds that low-dose and low-dose-rate radiation stimulates a set of biological responses in organisms that not only repair and defend against the radiogenic damage, but do so in excess of immediate need, so that they enhance protections even against other current and future sources of damage.[38]

According to Sacks et al., the BEIR VII report

> explicitly recognizes that a curved line fits better than a straight line for certain dose–response radiation data. Nevertheless the authors approximate that curve discontinuously by not one but two straight lines — one in the higher-dose region and a different one with a lower slope tangent to the lower-dose region — based on the use of a device called the dose and dose rate effectiveness factor (DDREF). This provides a means of modifying the linear model in order to preserve linearity.

Sacks et al. also claim that there is substantial evidence in favor of the notion that low doses of radiation protect against cancer:

> It had been found in the 1800s that some European uranium miners suffered higher rates of lung cancer, and it was found, through controlled studies, that the primary cause was high levels of radon in the mines. Many mines, however, have far lower levels of radon, and many uranium mines, replete with radon, in the U.S. and Europe are used as health spas where people go to sit for hours and days breathing in the radon in order to palliate their arthritic pain and gain other healthful results. Somewhere between the high levels of radon found in some of the European mines and other mines and places, there must be a threshold above which the effect is harmful and below which it is healthful".[39]

---

36 See for instance the 2018 exchange between Duncan et al. ("Radiation dose does matter: Mechanistic insights into DNA damage and repair support the linear no-threshold model of low-dose radiation health risks", *Journal of Nuclear Medicine* 59(7), 1014–1016) and Siegel et al. ("There is no evidence to support the linear no-threshold model of radiation carcinogenesis", *Journal of Nuclear Medicine* 59(12), 1918).

37 Sacks et al. (2016), "Epidemiology without biology: False paradigms, unfounded assumptions, and specious statistics in radiation science (with commentaries by Inge Schmitz-Feuerhake and Christopher Busby and a reply by the authors)", *Biological Theory* 11, 69–101.

38 Sacks et al. (2016), "Epidemiology without biology".

39 Sacks et al. (2016), "Epidemiology without biology", 78.

The paper by Sacks et al. does not provide any reference backing these claims.

Hormesis

Hormesis has been defined in a variety of ways, for instance as "any physiological effect that occurs at low doses which cannot be anticipated by extrapolating from toxic effects noted at high doses";[40] or as a biphasic dose response to an agent that at a low dose generates stimulation or beneficial effect and a high dose inhibitory or toxic effect;[41] much more broadly, hormesis has been defined as an "adaptive response characterized by biphasic dose responses of generally similar quantitative features with respect to amplitude and range of the stimulatory response that are either directly induced (...) or the result of compensatory biological processes following an initial disruption in homeostasis".[42] Ethanol has been posed as a typical example of hormesis, because moderate drinking is — allegedly — associated with lower risks of heart disease and other ailments, whereas heavy drinking is associated with higher risks.

Authors who defend the notion of hormesis have claimed that humans exhibit beneficial or "adaptive responses to low doses of neurotoxins" and carcinogens,[43] such as cadmium, dioxins, and ionizing radiation. This alleged beneficial response would be "generalizable across biological model, endpoint measured, and chemical class".[44] Furthermore, because "a strong case can be made for the use of hormesis as a default assumption in the risk-assessment", many low-dose chemical and radiation risks can be deregulated.[45]

Since the 1990s, the suggestion that hormesis could and should be used as the principal dose-response default assumption for purposes of understanding the biological action of physical or chemical agents or, most important, for regulatory purposes, has been opposed by authors who refer to major problems

---

40 Sagan (1987), "What is hormesis and why haven't we heard about it before?" *Health Physics* 52, 521–525.

41 Mattson (2008), "Hormesis defined", *Ageing Research Reviews* (1), 1–7.

42 Calabrese & Baldwin (2002), "Defining hormesis", *Human & Experimental Toxicology* 21(2), 91–97.

43 Calabrese (2008), "Astrocytes — Adaptive responses to low doses of neurotoxins", *Critical Reviews in Toxicology* 38(5), 463–471.

44 Calabrese (2005), "Historical blunders: How toxicology got the dose-response relationship half right", *Cellular and Molecular Biology* 51(7), 643–654.

45 Calabrese & Baldwin (2001), "Hormesis: A generalizable and unifying hypothesis", *Critical Reviews in Toxicology* 31(4–5), 353–424.

posed by the concept.[46] In general, it is accepted that some physical or chemical agents may have beneficial effects at low doses, but incorporating these effects into risk assessment ignores well-established notions related to exposure and human susceptibility, so that the application of hormesis in assessments of physical or chemical risks for regulatory purposes would not be at all sound.[47] Some of the problems cited to reject the applicability of hormesis as basic model to understand the interaction of physical agents or chemicals with animals or humans are the lack of data on repeatability of hormetic phenomena; the observation that many dose-response curves are not hormetic, so that hormesis cannot be generalized; and the fact that the mechanisms explaining hormesis as a phenomenon are not understood at a rigorous scientific level — compared, for instance, with models of pharmacological or toxicological dose-response such as the theories of Michaelis-Menten, receptor-ligand binding, single and multiple hit models, or the Moolgavkar-Knudson carcinogenesis model.[48] Overall, the definition of hormesis and the claims of its generalizability have been strongly disputed and remain largely problematic, as general mechanisms proposed for hormesis appear more speculative than driven by empirical evidence, and similarities to other biological phenomena do not permit direct borrowing in term of a plausible mechanism of action. It is indeed unlikely that a beneficial effect of a low-dose toxic on a specific end point can be useful to characterize agents that generate a variety of toxic effects in multiple organs and through multiple mechanisms.[49] For instance, it could be that moderate drinking reduces the risk of heart disease but raises the risk of breast cancer. In a recent paper Andrea Dei[50] elaborates on the links between hormesis and homeopathy from a sympathetic viewpoint that apparently intends to enhance the credibility of both notions. Probably, though, for more than one reader it will have the opposite effect. As explained by Kristin Shrader-Frechette, many important scientific bodies have produced statements that direct or indirectly represent pronouncements

---

46 Shrader-Frechette (2008), "Ideological toxicology: Invalid logic, science, ethics about low-dose pollution", *Human & Experimental Toxicology* 27(8), 647–657.

47 Axelrod et al. (2004), "Hormesis — An inappropriate extrapolation from the specific to the universal", *International Journal of Occupational and Environmental Health* 10(3), 335–339; Elliott (2000), "A case for caution: An evaluation of Calabrese and Baldwin's studies of chemical hormesis", *Risk* 11(2), 176–196.

48 Kitchin & Drane (2005), "A critique of the use of hormesis in risk assessment", *Human & Experimental Toxicology* 24, 249–253

49 Mushak (2007), "Hormesis and its place in nonmonotonic dose-response relationships: Some scientific reality checks", *Environmental Health Perspectives* 15(4), 500–506.

50 Dei (2017), "Hormesis and homeopathy — Toward a new self-consciousness", *Dose-Response* 15(4), 1–4.

against hormesis; thus the US National Research Council stated in 2004 that pesticide manufacturers and other interested parties have provided funding for studies trying to justify the reduction or elimination of chemical-safety standards — even though such deregulation is not scientifically defensible — and in 2006 the NRC also stated that available information does not support the contention that low levels of ionizing radiation have a beneficial effect.[51] Leaving aside chemical agents and focusing specifically on radiation, arguments supporting the view that sufficiently small doses of radiation induce no increase in cancer risk — i.e. a dose threshold — or a reduction in cancer risk — i.e. hormesis — were rejected by qualified bodies such as UNSCEAR and the National Radiological Protection Board of the UK.[52]

Probably the most prominent promoter of the hormesis notion is University of Massachusetts toxicologist Edward J. Calabrese.[53] Calabrese refers to himself in third person in his CV,[54] as follows:

> Over the past 20 years Professor Calabrese has redirected his research to understanding the nature of the dose response in the low dose zone and underlying adaptive explanatory mechanisms. Of particular note is that this research has led to important discoveries which indicate that the most fundamental dose response in toxicology and pharmacology is the hormetic-biphasic dose response relationship. These observations are leading to a major transformation in improving drug discovery, development, and in the efficiency of the clinical trial, as well as the scientific foundations for risk assessment and environmental regulation for radiation and chemicals.

---

51 Shrader-Frechette (2012), "Research integrity and conflicts of interest: The case of unethical research-misconduct charges filed by Edward Calabrese", *Accountability in Research* 19(4), 220 – 242.

52 UNSCEAR (1993), *Sources, and effects of ionizing radiation: United Nations Scientific Committee on the Effects of Atomic Radiation 1993 Report to the General Assembly, with annexes*, Annex G; Cox et al. (1995), *Risk of radiation-induced cancer at low doses and low dose rates for radiation protection purposes.*

53 Calabrese & Baldwin (1999), "The marginalization of hormesis", *Toxicological Pathology* 27(2), 187–194; Calabrese & Baldwin (2001), "The frequency of U-shaped dose responses in the toxicological literature", *Toxicological Sciences* 62(2), 330–338; Calabrese & Baldwin (2003), "Toxicology rethinks its central belief", *Nature* 421(6924), 691–692. Perhaps Linda A. Baldwin should be cited as the second most prominent defender of hormesis, as she has coauthored with Calabrese some 130 papers, which would not be exaggerated to say are most if not all of them about hormesis.

54 Dated January 2021 and downloaded in February 2022 from www.umass.edu/sphhs/person/edward-j-calabrese.

According to Calabrese, hormesis is not only the most fundamental dose-response relationship in toxicology and pharmacology, but also the key notion to explain the mechanism of pharmacological action of most anxiolytic, antiseizure drugs, drugs to improve memory, drugs for Alzheimer, and numerous other classes of drugs.[55] Calabrese's publications, numbering over 900, are to a large extent on hormesis and closely related fields. Despite his views are largely contested in the field and his notions on hormesis have been repeatedly rejected by scientific bodies and regulatory institutions, Calabrese has occupied important editorial roles in the field of toxicology. Among many other editorial jobs, he was the editor-in-chief of the journals *Human and Ecological Risk Assessment,* and *Non-linearity in Biology, Toxicology, and Medicine.* When this journal changed its name in 2005 to *Dose-Response*, Calabrese continued as editor-in-chief, to the present.[56]

Dose-Response, the journal edited by Calabrese, has published papers "demonstrating" the overestimation of Chernobyl consequences, for instance regarding the carcinogenic action of radioactive iodine, as well as other supposed weaknesses of investigations finding significant health consequences of the Chernobyl fallout.[57] *Dose-Response* has also published papers that present evidence from Chernobyl studies supposedly showing that the LNT model is wrong and that hormesis has been found in areas close to Chernobyl in which cesium-137 and other radioisotopes from the nuclear disaster have created low-dose radioactivity conditions since 1986.[58]

On August 23, 2011 Calabrese filed research misconduct charges against Kristin Shrader-Frechette, professor of biology and philosophy at Notre Dame University who had disputed in peer-reviewed publications Calabrese's claims on hormesis. Shrader-Frechette had argued that the notion that hormesis is a generalizable mechanism of interaction between physicochemical agents and living beings was based on several logical fallacies. In his charges against Shrader-Frechette, Calabrese claimed that she was guilty of "falsification of the research

---

55 Calabrese (2010), "Hormesis: Calabrese responds," *Environmental Health Perspectives* 118(4), 153–154. Note that drugs to improve memory or for treating Alzheimer disease are for the moment (but Calabrese was writing in 2010 or earlier) no more than a desire.
56 The number of publications and positions as editor-in-chief of journals according to his CV.
57 Jargin (2011), "Thyroid cancer after Chernobyl: Obfuscated truth", *Dose-Response* 9, 471–476; Jargin (2014), "On the radiation-leukemia dose-response relationship among recovery workers after the Chernobyl accident", *Dose-Response* 12(1), 162–165.
58 Jaworowski (2010), "Observations on the Chernobyl disaster and LNT", *Dose-Response* 8(2), 148–171; Rodgers & Holmes (2008), "Radio-adaptive response to environmental exposures at Chernobyl", *Dose-Response* 6(2), 209–221.

record by not interviewing or attempting to interview Calabrese" before publishing articles criticizing his publications as flawed science. Calabrese also claimed that Shrader-Frechette was guilty of misrepresentation, falsification and fabrication, because she stated in an article that Calabrese appeared to have more than $3,000,000 in funding from undisclosed sources, though he was mandated to disclose funding sources by university regulations. Calabrese also alleged that Shrader-Frechette was guilty of falsification of Calabrese's research methods because she argued that Calabrese routinely ignored or glossed over major methodological issues like statistical power, statistical significance, data variability and endpoint measurement among others, raising important questions about the scientific validity of his claims. The thick binder of allegations of Calabrese against Shrader-Frechette, as thick as a textbook of internal medicine and obviously prepared, at great expense, by one or more attorneys, not Calabrese alone, was obviously intended to destroy her career, reputation, and employment. Calabrese did not reveal who funded his research misconduct attack on Shrader-Frechette, but she revealed that in the past, Calabrese's contract funding had come from companies such as Atlantic Richfield Oil, BASF (the world's largest chemicals producer), Bayer Chemical, Chemical Manufacturers Association, Dow, Exxon, Reynolds Metals, Rohm and Haas Chemicals, Shell Chemical, Syngenta pesticides, Texas Institute for Advancement of Chemical Technology, and Union Carbide, all of whom would benefit financially from deregulation in the oil, chemical, and nuclear industries and from the acceptance of hormesis as a valid scientific concept that would raise questions about the validity of regulating chemicals and physical agents like radiation, especially at low levels of exposure. On November 28, 2011, after three months of assessment, the committee of the University of Notre Dame charged with the evaluation of the research misconduct allegations unanimously and fully exonerated Shrader-Frechette: "having conducted a close and careful examination, the Committee finds that the evidence does not support allegations of research misconduct.[59]

The CV of Edward Calabrese dated January 2021 does indeed include a long list of grants for the project BELLE (Biological Effects of Low-Level Exposures) as well as funding for projects on hormesis from a variety of corporations, with amounts of hundreds of thousands dollars per year during many years.[60]

---

59 Shrader-Frechette (2012), "Research integrity and conflicts of interest".

60 Overall, that Calabrese received "millions of dollars of special-interest funding for defending the oil, chemical, and nuclear industry" (as stated by Shrader-Frechette (2008), "Ideological toxicology") appears very consistent with the information in Calabrese's CV.

Hormesis promoters have often claimed that regulation of toxic exposures is useless, given the generally beneficial effects of low-dose exposures.[61] Since deregulation would save the oil, chemical, and nuclear industries significant money on pollution control, there appears to be an excellent rationale for financing hormesis research, and hormesis defenders, by these industries. *Critical Reviews in Toxicology*, the journal in which many of Calabrese's papers have appeared, is published in England by Informa UK Ltd, a for-profit company that claims to have as its driving purpose "to help businesses and professionals to learn more, know more and do more" and to be committed to a "positive impact that the knowledge and connections we deliver can create for our customers, markets and communities".[62] In brief, Informa UK Ltd is a marketing and PR tool and a journal like *Critical Reviews in Toxicology* fulfills an important role in that context, presenting as scientific information the business views of the industry.

Given current knowledge, the LNT model continues to be a very acceptable description and explanation of the effects of physical and chemical agents on living organisms. Perhaps additions like DREFs and DDREFs are needed to complement the LNT model, and perhaps the model will be further refined, modified, and even discarded in the future, when more is discovered about how low-level radiations interact with organisms. For now, it appears that supporters of hormesis, at least some of which have significant conflicts of interests, have come up against solid empirical research and credible interpretations based on the best data and theory available.

---

61 Calabrese & Baldwin (2001), "Hormesis: A generalizable...".
62 Informa Inc. website, www.informa.com/about-us/group-policies/, accessed February 2022.

Chapter 9
Conflicting results of investigations on exposures to low-dose ionizing radiation

Conflicting evaluations of the effect of low-dose ionizing radiation in official statements of national or international organizations no doubt reflect to a large extent the conflicting findings and interpretations of empirical investigations. But consensus views in official statements may also in turn influence empirical research, since results that do not fit previous expectations can be easily discarded as biased.

Since the 1990s, investigations of the health effects of specific instances in which low-level radiation was suspected or certain have often been controversial and different researchers have sometimes interpreted the same results differently. Thus, epidemiologists studying the incidence of cancer after the 1979 accident in the nuclear plant of Three Mile Island, close to Harrisburg, Pennsylvania, agreed on the findings of an increase in cancer incidence after the accident, but disagreed on whether this could be reasonably interpreted as a causal effect of the released radiation. Some viewed the data as indicative of a carcinogenic effect of the radiation presumably received from the accident, while others interpreted the evidence as insufficient to demonstrate an influence of the released radioactivity on the cancer risk during the period of follow-up.[1] A major issue in this controversy was the estimation of the amount of radiation received after the accident by persons living near Three Mile Island.

In the case of Three Mile Island the controversy involved different groups of researchers who had different views on the amount of radiation that had been received by the residents in the area of fallout. In contrast, in investigations

---

[1] Hatch et al. (1990), "Cancer near the Three Mile Island nuclear plant: Radiation emissions", *American Journal of Epidemiology* 132(3), 392–412; Hatch et al. (1991), "Cancer rates after the Three Mile Island nuclear accident and proximity of residence to the plant", *American Journal of Public Health* 81(6), 719–724; Wing et al. (1997), "A reevaluation of cancer incidence near the Three Mile Island nuclear plant: the collision of evidence and assumptions", *Environmental Health Perspectives* 105(1), 52–57; Hatch et al. (1997), "Comments on 'A Reevaluation of Cancer Incidence near the Three Mile Island Nuclear Plant'", *Environmental Health Perspectives* 105(1), 12; Talbott et al. (2000a), "Mortality among the residents of the Three Mile Island accident area: 1979–1992", *Environmental Health Perspectives* 108, 545–552; Wing & Richardson (2000), "Collision of evidence and assumptions: TMI déjà view", *Environmental Health Perspectives* 108(12), A546-A547; Talbott et al. (2000b), "Re: 'Collision of Evidence and assumptions: TMI Déjà View'" *Environmental Health Perspectives* 108, 12.

https://doi.org/10.1515/9783110761788-013

on the potential carcinogenic effects of the fallout from Chernobyl on cancer incidence in Sweden, varying results came mostly from the same researchers who focused on levels of cesium-137 from the fallout as predictors of cancer incidence. This is something that is worth to be told with some detail, as it is instructive on how scientific knowledge advances sometimes in a quite tortuous manner.

Because a substantial amount (usually estimated in 5%) of the total fallout of cesium-137 from Chernobyl fell on Sweden, it is not surprising that Swedish authors were soon actively investigating the possible harmful effects of this radioactive deposition. In a study published in 2004, Martin Tondell and four other authors analyzed the incidence of cancer in 1988–1996 in relation to the fallout of caesium-137.[2] A total of 450 parishes in northern Sweden were categorized in six levels of caesium-137 deposition, the lowest deposition category defined as less than 3 kilobecquerel per square meter (kBq/m^2), and the other categories in order of increasing exposure, 3–29, 30–39, 40–59, 60–79, until the highest exposure category, 80–120 kBq/m^2. All individuals aged 60 years or less living in these parishes between 1986 and 1987 conformed a study cohort of over a million people in which some 22,000 incident cancer cases were diagnosed in 1988–1996. Taking age, population density, lung cancer incidence in 1988–1996, and total cancer incidence in 1986–1987 by municipality as potential confounders, the adjusted relative risks for the deposition categories were 1.00 (by definition, in the reference group with less than 3 kBq/m^2), and 1.05, 1.03, 1.08, 1.10, and 1.21 respectively in the other five groups, ordered by increasing level of exposure. The excess relative risk was 0.11 per 100 kBq/m^2, with a 95% confidence interval from 0.03 to 0.20. The authors interpreted that the light increase in total cancer incidence occurred in northern Sweden after the Chernobyl accident seems to be causally linked to the exposure to radiation unless attributable to chance or remaining uncontrolled confounding factors.

Two years later, in 2006, an almost identical group of authors also led by Tondel analyzed the incidence of malignancies in Sweden by studying a cohort of over a million residents of ages 60 or less in 1986 who lived in any of the 8 counties of Sweden with the highest fallout of caesium-137.[3] Using the dwelling coordinates, and a digital map on caesium-137, the exposure of each individual was estimated. During the follow-up, 1988–1999, 33,851 malignancies were diagnosed. The level of exposure to ionized radiation was categorized in nanograys

---

2 Tondel et al. (2004), "Increase of regional total cancer incidence in north Sweden due to the Chernobyl accident?", *Journal of Epidemiology & Community Health* 58, 1011.

3 Tondel et al. (2006), "Increased incidence of malignancies in Sweden after the Chernobyl accident — A promoting effect?", *American Journal of Industrial Medicine* 49(3), 159–168.

per hour (nGy/hr) in the following categories: 0 – 8 (reference), 9 – 23, 24 – 43, 44 – 66, 67 – 84, and 85 nGy/hr. The corresponding adjusted incidence rate ratios for total malignancies during follow-up in the six exposure groups ordered by increasing level of radiation exposure were 1.000 (by definition), 0.997, 1.072, 1.114, 1.068, and 1.125, respectively (i. e., the risk of cancer in the group of highest exposure was 12.5 % higher than in the reference group of lowest exposure). The authors concluded that their findings revealed an increased incidence of total malignancies possibly related to the fallout from the Chernobyl disaster.

Eight years later, in 2014 a new investigation was published on the potential relationship between cancer incidence in northern Sweden and the Chernobyl fallout, authored by Hassan Alinaghizadeh, Martin Tondel, and Robert Wålinder. Of this three authors, only Tondel had been an author — the first one — of the two previous papers.[4] The relation between exposure to deposition of cesium-137 and cancer incidence after the Chernobyl fallout was investigated in the nine northernmost counties of Sweden, where 2.2 million inhabitants lived in 1986. The level of radioactivity was estimated for each county and for each of the 612 parishes included in these 9 counties from the maps of fallout in 1986. Diagnoses of cancer from 1980 to 2009 amounted to 273,222 cases. Age-adjusted incidence rate ratios, stratified by gender, were calculated with Poisson regression in two cohorts corresponding to the pre-Chernobyl and the post-Chernobyl periods, 1980 – 1985 and 1986 – 2009, respectively. No obvious exposure-response pattern was found in the age-adjusted total cancer incidence rate ratios and an association between fallout and cancer incidence that was found was considered spurious as it was seen that areas with the lowest incidence of cancer before the accident had the lowest fallout of cesium-137. A secular trend with an increase in age-standardized incidence of cancer in both genders from 1980 to 2009, was statistically significant only in females and stronger and significant for both genders in the general Swedish population. The authors concluded that using both high quality cancer registry data and high-resolution exposure maps of radioactive deposition, it was not possible to distinguish an effect of such deposition on cancer incidence after the Chernobyl accident in Sweden. The association found in the two previous Swedish studies was thus spurious, they concluded, and perhaps due to confounding from unadjusted regional differences in the incidence of cancer before the accident.

Reading these papers was quite puzzling and I decided to attempt to get some clarification from the authors, so I emailed them. In a brief email I ex-

---

4 Alinaghizadeh et al. (2014), "Cancer incidence in northern Sweden before and after the Chernobyl nuclear power plant accident", *Radiation & Environmental Biophysics* 53, 495 – 504.

pressed my surprise about the fact that while the two papers published in 2004 and 2006 in which Tondel was the first author had both accepted, with proper qualifications, the evidence as showing a causal link between the Chernobyl fallout in Sweden and the subsequent incidence of cancer, the 2014 paper in which Alinaghizadeh was first author and Tondel the second one explicitly rejected this causal link as unsupported by the data. I also explained in my email my surprise about the fact that the other authors of the 2004 and 2006 papers were not authors of the 2014 paper and asked whether perhaps there had been disagreements about the content of that paper.

A few days later, in March 20, 2020, I received a kind email from Robert Wålinder. He wrote that you must "not be too categorical when doing epidemiological studies. Changing your view is sometimes good. But the thing is that we haven't got the final answer yet." He said that more papers where in the pipeline and referred to me to an article that had been published in 2016, authored by Alinaghizadeh, Wålinder, Vingård, and Tondel.[5]

In this 2016 paper it was stated that in the previous study of 2014 it had not been possible to establish an exposure–response pattern perhaps because the study had an ecological design in which the exposure had been measured at the level of geographical units. Indeed, the fallout of cesium-137 after Chernobyl had been in Sweden quite irregular because it rained during the first week after the accident. Therefore, an ecological study using mean values at the county, municipality or parish level necessarily will have less precision in detecting an association between the level of exposure to radionuclides and cancer. Thus, in the new study, Alinaghizadeh et al. said, they had decided to restrict the study population to the counties most affected by Chernobyl fallout in 1986 and to increase the precision of the exposure assessment by estimating individual exposures for all members of the cohort of some 700,000 persons living in the three counties most contaminated in Sweden by cesium-137 from Chernobyl. Exposure was estimated for each individual on the basis of location of residence each year between 1986 and 1990 and cesium-137 radioactivity as reported in the Geological Survey of Sweden. A total of 82,495 persons were diagnosed with cancer in this cohort in the years 1991–2010. In the statistical analysis the hazard of developing cancer was estimated with a Cox model in which the exposure was categorized in three groups and adjustment were included for age, sex, rural or non-rural residence, and pre-Chernobyl total cancer incidence. A exposure–

5 Alinaghizadeh et al. (2016), "Total cancer incidence in relation to ^{137}Cs fallout in the most contaminated counties in Sweden after the Chernobyl nuclear power plant accident: a register-based study", *BMJ Open* 6(12), e011924.

response pattern was found so that the hazard was the highest in the group of individuals more exposed (a hazard ratio of 1.06 compared to the hazard in the less exposed group), while the hazard was intermediate (hazard ratio of 1.04) in the individuals of intermediate exposure. Despite the pattern of relation between exposure and cancer incidence is clearly consistent with a causal effect, the authors judged the strength of the association to be too small as to infer with certainty a causal link.

It would be easy to discard the controversies on the importance of effects of low-level radiation from mines, nuclear plants, or nuclear disasters as purely ideological, driven by the researchers' previous beliefs. However, the case of the studies on cancer incidence in Sweden quite clearly illustrates how that would be an erroneous interpretation of the situation in a research area in which major scientific problems are still unsettled.

Chapter 10
Thyroid cancer caused by the Chernobyl fallout

Childhood thyroid cancer provides the best example of empirical research converging toward strong evidence of a causal link between exposure to low-dose ionizing radiation from fallout and appearance of cancer with a short-latency of 5 years or less. Knowledge of this causal link evolved in the scientific community in the 1990s through observations and epidemiological studies after Chernobyl, and represented a break with prior understanding based mostly on earlier studies of Japanese A-bomb survivors. At the time of the Chernobyl disaster thyroid cancer was not considered radiogenic, as it was known that using 131-iodine to treat Graves' disease in adults led to hypothyroidism, not to cancer, and in addition, previous studies of children exposed to ionizing radiation from A-bombs, medical X-rays, or radiotherapy had reported an increased incidence of thyroid cancer – but only with latencies of 10 years or more.[1] Thus when a few years after the Chernobyl disaster Soviet doctors started to talk about increasing cases of thyroid cancer in areas of Chernobyl fallout, their reports were received with significant skepticism. In 1991 the IAEA published a technical report noting that by the end of 1990, there had been 20 verified cases of thyroid cancer in children of the Soviet Socialist Republic of Ukraine, but 11 of these cases had been diagnosed in non-contaminated areas suggesting that these cancers were not connected to the Chernobyl fallout. In addition, the report plainly dismissed the idea that exposure had caused thyroid cancer by stating that most of the reports of thyroid cancer "were anecdotal in nature with little evidence relative to the population size and age composition from which the cases were derived."[2] An observer noted that "the mandate of the IAEA enjoins it to promote the peaceful use of nuclear technology, and this, together with its close links to the nuclear industry, would not make evidence of carcinogenic risks following a nuclear accident welcome news".[3]

Nine years after the Chernobyl disaster, a letter in the *BMJ*, the prestigious British medical journal, reported an incidence of childhood thyroid cancer in the region of Gomel in Belarus of 96.4 per million children below age 15, compared to a pre-Chernobyl incidence of childhood thyroid cancer of about 0.5

---

1 Williams (2002), "Cancer after nuclear fallout: lessons from the Chernobyl accident", *Nature Reviews — Cancer* 2(7), 543.
2 IAEA (1991), *The international Chernobyl Project: Assessment of radiological consequences and evaluation of protective measures — Report by an International Advisory Committee,* 388.
3 Baverstock & Williams (2006), "The Chernobyl accident 20 years on".

https://doi.org/10.1515/9783110761788-014

per million.[4] This is a relative risk of about 200, which means that virtually all cases of childhood thyroid cancer in the region can be attributed to the Chernobyl fallout.[5] Given the low levels of radiation supposedly received by the residents in the areas of Ukraine, Belarus and Russia where a high incidence of childhood thyroid cancer had been detected, the low carcinogenicity that radioactive iodine was assumed to have, and the short latency between the exposure and the appearance of these tumors, international agencies and many scientists were reluctant to acknowledge that the epidemic of thyroid cancer in children that was being reported could be linked to exposure to radiation from Chernobyl.[6] However, now the evidence was much more clear and preconceptions started to crumble. An independent epidemiological review concluded that the causal link between Chernobyl radiation and the epidemic of thyroid cancer in children was undeniable.[7] Then, in its 1996 report, IAEA recognized that by 1995 a sharp increase in thyroid cancer among children had been observed, which was "the only major public health impact from radiation exposure documented to date." About 800 cases in children under 15 years of age had been diagnosed in Belarus and northern Ukraine, with 3 children known to have died of cancer.[8] But the IAEA report mentioned that thyroid cancer can generally be successfully treated, that the incidence of thyroid cancer among children born more than 6 months after the accident had remained at the low levels expected in unexposed populations, which confirmed that the risk of thyroid cancer was only increased among those receiving high thyroid doses in 1986 and not among those exposed only to the continuing low levels of exposure since then. The report also acknowledged that in the long run an increase in the incidence of thyroid cancer in adults who received radiation doses as children *could occur*, with the total number of cases possibly in the order of a few thousands.

During the 1990s thyroid cancer became the most obvious and undeniable consequence of Chernobyl and thus the 2000 UNSCEAR report had to acknowledge the facts. But the report also referred to the influence of screening on the enhanced detection of cases, to uncertainties in the baseline rates used to quantify the magnitude of the increase in incidence, and to the short time lag between

4 Stsjazhko (1995), "Childhood thyroid cancer since accident at Chernobyl", *BMJ* 310(6982), 801.
5 Baverstock & Williams (2006), "The Chernobyl accident 20 years on: An assessment of the health consequences and the international response", *Environmental Health Perspectives* 114, 1312–1317.
6 Williams (2002), "Cancer after nuclear fallout".
7 Bard et al. (1997), "Chernobyl, 10 years after: Health consequences", *Epidemiologic Reviews* 19(2), 187–204.
8 IAEA (1996), *After Chernobyl: What do we really know?*

exposure and cases that was inconsistent with previous knowledge about thyroid cancer. Nevertheless, the report plainly asserted that there could be "no doubt about the relationship between the radioactive materials released from the Chernobyl accident and the unusually high number of thyroid cancers observed in the contaminated areas during the past 14 years".[9] An epidemiological review published in 2002 mentioned the reluctance of international bodies to acknowledge the link between Chernobyl and the epidemic of thyroid cancer and their attempt to attribute this epidemic to intense thyroid screening initiatives implemented after the Chernobyl accident, but concluded also that there was good evidence "to suggest that rates of thyroid cancer in children from the countries that were formally part of the Soviet Union have risen as a consequence of the Chernobyl accident".[10]

Early estimates by experts in radiation epidemiology had suggested that some 1500 added thyroid cancers could be caused by the radioactive iodine deposited by the Chernobyl fallout over a 30-year period.[11] In 1996 the IAEA report on Chernobyl referred to about 800 cases in children under age 15 already diagnosed, but this was just 10 years after the disaster. In 2006 the Chernobyl Forum stated that 4000 or 5000 cases of thyroid cancer had been diagnosed in Russian, Ukrainian and Belorussian children.[12] In 2011 Fred Mettler, leader of the medical research team of the Chernobyl Forum, stated that 7000 cases of thyroid cancer had occurred because of the Chernobyl fallout.[13] Five years later, in a 30-year summary update, WHO stated that by 2016 more than 11,000 thyroid cancer cases had been diagnosed in children and adolescents of the three affected countries.[14]

Epidemiological knowledge on Chernobyl-related thyroid cancer has been increasingly refined evolving from the early case reports and ecological studies to more rigorous investigations with individual-level estimates of exposure. For example, a cohort study of 12,514 individuals aged 18 or less on 26 April 1986 who resided in contaminated areas of Ukraine revealed a linear dose-response

9 UNSCEAR (2000), *Sources and effects of ionizing radiation: UNSCEAR 2000 Report to the General Assembly*, Annex J, 514.
10 Moysich et al. (2002), "Chernobyl-related ionising radiation exposure and cancer risk: An epidemiological review", *Lancet Oncology* 3(5), 269–279.
11 Fabrikant (1987), "The Chernobyl disaster: An international perspective", *Industrial Crisis Quarterly* 1(4), 2–12.
12 Chernobyl Forum: 2003–2005 (2006), *Chernobyl's legacy: Health, environmental and socioeconomic impacts, and recommendations to the governments of Belarus, the Russian Federation and Ukraine*.
13 Joyce (2011), "WBUR News: Challenges loom large, 25 years after Chernobyl" (April 26).
14 WHO (2016), "1986–2016: Chernobyl at 30 – An update".

relationship between the individual iodine-131 thyroid dose and the risk of thyroid cancer;[15] this risk persisted for two decades after exposure, with no evidence of decrease during the observation period. Unfortunately, this was not consistent with early assurances that had been given after the Chernobyl accident that, because of the short half-life of radioactive iodine, any harmful effect of the Chernobyl deposition of this isotope would decline quickly in months or just a few years.

Overall, today there is strong consensus that the exposure to ionizing radiation from the Chernobyl accident has increased the incidence of thyroid cancers dramatically in those who were children and were exposed to the fallout, with higher risk the younger the age of exposure.[16] But investigations of thyroid cancer risk in cohorts of liquidators exposed as adults suggest that similar effects may be present in adults.[17] There are also reports from countries outside the area of the old USSR showing rising trends of thyroid cancer. For example, in a paper published in 2004 epidemiologists in Poland noted that in recent years a slightly increased incidence of thyroid had been observed in the population aged 15 years or less, and argued that the increase could have been caused by the radiation from Chernobyl.[18] Increasing rates of thyroid cancer in other countries over the past decades[19] also suggest possible links to Chernobyl; however, these trends are also compatible with effects of other sources of low-dose ionizing radiation such as nuclear tests and industrial and medical uses of radionuclides, X-rays and other forms of ionizing radiation which have also increased over time.[20]

---

15 Brenner et al. (2012), "I-131 dose response for incident thyroid cancers in Ukraine related to the Chornobyl accident", *Environmental Health Perspectives* 119(8), A332.
16 Cardis et al. (2006), "Cancer consequences of the Chernobyl accident: 20 years on", *Journal of Radiological Protection* 26(2), 127–140; Ricarte-Filho et al. (2013), "Identification of kinase fusion oncogenes in post-Chernobyl radiation-induced thyroid cancers", *Journal of Clinical Investigation* 123(11), 4935–4944.
17 Hatch & Cardis (2017), "Somatic health effects of Chernobyl: 30 years on", *European Journal of Epidemiology* 32(12), 1047–1054.
18 Roszkowska & Goryński (2004) ["Thyroid cancer in Poland in 1980–2000"] [in Polish], *Przegląd Epidemiologiczny* 58(2), 369–376.
19 Lim et al. (2017), "Trends in thyroid cancer incidence and mortality in the United States, 1974–2013", *JAMA* 317(13), 1338–1348; Tondel et al. (2004), "Increase of regional total cancer incidence in north Sweden due to the Chernobyl accident?", *Journal of Epidemiology & Community Health* 58, 1011.
20 Brown (2019), *Manual for survival – A Chernobyl guide to the future*, 311–312.

Chapter 11
Post-Chernobyl non-thyroid malignancies and other health effects

During the present century, the view that early projections of the health impact of the Chernobyl disaster were overly optimistic has been gaining weight. Early projections were often based on the idea that low-dose radiation was mostly innocuous, though in the long run it could have some carcinogenic effects on the thyroid and the blood-producing organs. But that was it. As thyroid cancer is generally treatable and curable, only a few thousand cancer deaths, mostly from leukemia over a period of many decades, were expected from the Chernobyl accident. Thus the impact would be small, compared to the health effects of say, smoking, epidemics of infectious diseases like AIDS, or particulate atmospheric pollution causing hundreds of thousands or even million annual deaths.

This optimistic view of the limited harmful effects of the Chernobyl disaster was evident in the 2000 UNSCEAR report which noted that despite the fact that leukemia was known to be one of the early carcinogenic effects of ionizing radiation with a latency period of only a few years, investigations of leukemia risk in populations exposed to the Chernobyl fallout had provided no evidence of increased leukemia among liquidators or among residents of contaminated areas.[1] Reviews of the health effects of Chernobyl published in the scientific literature in the 1990s or in the first decade of the present century generally supported this view, as overall it was concluded that for childhood thyroid cancer the evidence of a causal link with the Chernobyl disaster was strong, but for leukemia, other cancers or other disorders, no evidence of a link with Chernobyl radiation was found.[2] Early suspicions of the carcinogenic effects of the Chernobyl fallout were often rejected as exaggerated, or inconsistent with established knowledge, or unsound on the basis of a reexamination of the data. Thus, for instance, an early suspicion of post-Chernobyl carcinogenic effects of fallout

---

1 UNSCEAR (2000), *Sources and effects of ionizing radiation: UNSCEAR 2000 Report to the General Assembly*, Annex J, 507.
2 Bard et al. (1997), "Chernobyl, 10 years after: Health consequences", *Epidemiologic Reviews* 19(2), 187–204; Moysich et al. (2002), "Chernobyl-related ionising radiation exposure and cancer risk: An epidemiological review", *Lancet Oncology*, 3(5), 269–279; Cardis et al. (2006), "Cancer consequences of the Chernobyl accident: 20 years on", *Journal of Radiological Protection* 26(2), 127–140.

https://doi.org/10.1515/9783110761788-015

on childhood neuroblastomas in Germany was ruled out by a properly done case-control study.[3]

When early studies of Chernobyl liquidators or residents in areas highly exposed to the Chernobyl fallout detected statistically insignificant increases of other cancer risks, or even when statistically significant effects were found, inconsistency with previous knowledge based on the Japanese A-bomb survivors exposed at low doses was considered a good reason to attribute the increased incidence of cancer to bias in sampling, overdetection of clinically latent cases due to post-Chernobyl screening, or other reasons. This is what apparently occurred in the case of a study of childhood leukemia cases and controls in Russia, Belarus and Ukraine authored in 2005 by researchers of the International Consortium for Research on the Health Effects of Radiation, which had funding from the US Office of Naval Research. Despite quite low estimated radiation doses received by the study participants, there was an overall statistically significant increase in leukemia risk, most evident in Ukraine, associated with higher radiation dose.[4] The findings suggested that prolonged exposure to very low radiation doses may increase leukemia risk as much as or even more than acute exposure, but since this was inconsistent with previous views in the scientific literature, the large excess risks and significant dose–response observed was attributed by the authors to an overestimation of risk in Ukraine. The authors concluded that there was "no convincing evidence of an increased risk of childhood leukaemia as a result of exposure to Chernobyl radiation".

Other authors were more cautious in interpreting results that were not statistically significant but nevertheless showed increases in risk. Two linked studies of non-thyroid cancer in Ukrainian and Belarussian individuals exposed in childhood to Chernobyl fallout found an increase in the incidence of non-thyroid solid cancer, lymphoma or leukemia that was substantial but was not statistically significant.[5] The circumspect investigators concluded that these results were suggestive of effects on solid cancers despite the lack of statistical significance, and that the long latency of effect on solid cancers may have affected the ability

---

3 Michaelis et al. (1996), "Case-control study of neuroblastoma in west-Germany after the Chernobyl accident", *Klinische Pädiatrie* 208(4), 172–178.
4 Davis et al. (2005), "Childhood leukaemia in Belarus, Russia, and Ukraine following the Chernobyl power station accident: Results from an international collaborative population-based case–control study", *International Journal of Epidemiology* 35(2), 386–396.
5 Hatch et al. (2015), "Non-thyroid cancer in Northern Ukraine in the post-Chernobyl period: Short report", *Cancer Epidemiology* 39(3), 279–283; Ostroumova et al. (2016), "Non-thyroid cancer incidence in Belarusian residents exposed to Chernobyl fallout in childhood and adolescence: Standardized incidence ratio analysis, 1997–2011", *Environmental Research* 147, 44–49.

to reveal stronger or statistically significant associations. A basic principle of science is that no significant evidence does not in any way equals evidence of no effect.[6] However, this is often forgotten, our preconceptions are usually reinforced by the lack of evidence against them.

Inconsistencies in early results, very often determined by small sample sizes and the associated lack of statistical power, short follow-up periods, poor dosimetric methods, and other technical problems have been often solved in subsequent investigations. Overall, during the present century, research on Chernobyl and other cases of low-dose exposure has confirmed many hypotheses regarding radiation exposures that had been either dismissed or merely suggested by previous studies.

General effects of low dose ionizing radiation from Chernobyl fallout on the human organism and particularly on the nervous system are suggested by some papers published during the present century in economic journals. Ukrainian data from a panel survey of approximately 8800 individuals aged 16 and over revealed a positive association between the radiation dose received by an area and the perception of poor health by the individuals who had been exposed in that area. The authors of the study concluded that their findings provided suggestive evidence that those who lived in areas more exposed to Chernobyl-induced radiation have significantly lower levels of labour market performance 20 years on.[7] With data from the 2003–2008 waves of the Belarusian Household Survey of Income and Expenditure it was found that young individuals who came from the most contaminated areas of Belarus had worse health and lower probability of holding a university degree and being employed, and had lower wages compared to those who came from less contaminated areas.[8] Further away from Chernobyl, Swedish authors found that the prenatal exposure to Chernobyl fallout had effects on cognitive ability, with the students born in regions of Sweden with higher fallout performing worse in secondary school, in mathematics in particular, than those who were born in regions where the fallout had been low. The authors concluded that from a public health perspective,

6 Altman & Bland (1995), "Absence of evidence is not evidence of absence", *BMJ* 326(7401), 1267.
7 Lehmann & Wadsworth (2011), "The impact of Chernobyl on health and labour market performance", *Journal of Health Economics* 30(5), 843–857.
8 Yemelyanau et al. (2012), "Evidence from the Chernobyl Nuclear Accident: The Effect on Health, Education, and Labor Market Outcomes in Belarus", *Journal of Labor Research* 33(1), 1–20.

their findings suggested "that cognitive ability is compromised at radiation doses currently considered harmless".[9]

In 2016, at the Gilbert W. Beebe symposium "30 years after the Chernobyl accident: Current and future studies on radiation health effects", several peer reviewed studies showing links between radiation exposures related to Chernobyl and various health outcomes were presented.[10] In the Ukrainian cohort of liquidators Zablotska and colleagues had found evidence of a significant linear dose-response relationship for all types of leukemia, with the surprising finding of a non statistically significant dose-response association of similar magnitude for both chronic lymphocytic leukemia (CLL) and non-CLL. Since CLL had been previously judged to be clearly unrelated to ionizing radiation, this was an obvious challenge to prior conclusions from studies in Japanese A-bomb survivors.[11] Increases of both types of leukemia that were not statistically significant have been also reported in cohorts of liquidators in Russia, Belarus, and the Baltic countries, along with a statistically significant dose-dependent increase in non-Hodgkin lymphoma. A study in the cohort of liquidators found a strong dose-response relationship between the risk of developing thyroid cancer and the individual dose to the thyroid from external radiation and from iodine-131. In this case the estimates of ERR per 100 mSv were ten times bigger than the estimates reported in the Japanese A-bomb survivors exposed in adulthood.[12] Studies of liquidators from Ukraine, Russia, and the Baltic countries have provided evidence that this group of adults, mostly young males when first exposed to the Chernobyl radiation, has experienced a dose-related incidence of malignancies, including leukemia, non-Hodgkin lymphoma, thyroid cancer, and possibly multiple myeloma, and other types of neoplasm.[13]

Regarding CVD risks, it was reported at the Beebe Symposium that updated analyses of observations in Russian liquidators had revealed a dose-response relationship between estimated radiation received after Chernobyl and cerebrovas-

---

9 Almond & Palme (2009), "Chernobyl's subclinical legacy: Prenatal exposure to radioactive fallout and school outcomes in Sweden", *Quarterly Journal of Economics* 124(4), 1729–1772.
10 Samet et al. (2018), "Gilbert W. Beebe Symposium on 30 Years after the Chernobyl Accident: Current and Future Studies on Radiation Health Effects", *Radiation Research* 189(1), 5–18.
11 Zablotska et al. (2013), "Radiation and the risk of chronic lymphocytic and other leukemias among Chornobyl cleanup workers", *Environmental Health Perspectives* 121(1), 59–65; Ad hoc Working Group, US Department of Health & Human Services, Public Health Service (1985), *Report of the NIH ad hoc working group to develop radioepidemiological tables*.
12 Kesminiene et al. (2012), "Risk of thyroid cancer among Chernobyl liquidators", *Radiation Research* 178(5), 425–436, see particularly Table 6.
13 Hatch & Cardis (2017), "Somatic health effects of Chernobyl: 30 years on", *European Journal of Epidemiology* 32(17), 1047–1054.

cular outcomes.[14] This was in line with the UNSCEAR report of 2008 in which the CVD effects of the Chernobyl fallout had been reviewed and a dose-response relationship had been identified for various CVD end points in Russian liquidators.[15] Considering the low radiation doses that these liquidators had received, these CVD disorders and the increased incidence of solid cancers found in these workers were unexpected considering previous knowledge.

In what could be a revindication of early findings by Soviet researchers on the effects of the Chernobyl fallout on the health of mothers and newborns in contaminated areas of Belarus and Ukraine,[16] findings that were quite drastically dismissed by French authors in the 1990s,[17] preliminary results presented at the Beebe Symposium by Maureen Hatch suggested a dose-related reduction in head circumference of newborns exposed in utero, with the greatest reductions for those exposed early in gestation.[18] Increased risks of breast cancer, endocrine diseases, and CVD mortality, suggesting a causal impact of the Chernobyl fallout, have been found among residents of contaminated areas in Ukraine.[19] In a recently published study childhood leukemia during the post-Chernobyl period was more frequent in areas more contaminated by radiation.[20] Of course, many of these studies have weaknesses and need to be confirmed by further investigations, but what these investigations suggest is an impact of the Chernobyl fallout on the general level of health of the population exposed to low doses that was not even suspected considering the knowledge based on studies of Japanese survivors of the atomic bombing. Given the high prevalence and incidence of CVD and its role as a major cause of ill health and death in all countries, if confirmed

---

14 Kashcheev et al. (2015), Incidence and mortality of solid cancer among emergency workers of the Chernobyl accident: Assessment of radiation risks for the follow-up period of 1992–2009", *Radiation & Environmental Biophysics* 54(1), 13–23.

15 UNSCEAR (2008), "The Chernobyl accident: UNSCEAR's assessments of the radiation effects", accessed April 2020.

16 Kulakov et al. (1993), "Female reproductive function in areas affected by radiation after the Chernobyl power station accident", *Environmental Health Perspectives* 101, 117–123.

17 Bard et al. (1997), "Chernobyl, 10 years after: Health consequences", *Epidemiologic Reviews* 19(2), 187–204.

18 Samet et al. (2018), "Gilbert W. Beebe Symposium".

19 Pukkala et al. (2006), "Breast cancer in Belarus and Ukraine after the Chernobyl accident", *International Journal of Cancer* 119(3), 651–658.

20 Liubarets et al. (2019), "Childhood leukemia in Ukraine after the Chornobyl accident", *Radiation & Environmental Biophysics* 58(4), 553–562.

the effects of low-dose radiation on CVD are specially important from a public health perspective.[21]

Many effects of radiation take a long time to develop. As very eloquently explained by Williams and Baverstock, 20 years after the nuclear bombing of Japan

> the Atomic Bomb Casualty Commission reported significant increases in the incidence of just two cancers — thyroid cancer and leukaemia. It was another decade before a significant increase in other cancers was reported. Almost 45 years after the bombs, unexpected and significant increases in a range of non-cancer diseases, including heart disease, were found. And nearly 50 years after exposure, significant increases were reported for ten different cancers, with risks approximately doubled for colon, lung, breast, ovary and bladder tumours.[22]

Over time, studies of the effects of the Chernobyl fallout have produced increasingly strong evidence that has challenged previous views on radiobiology and radioepidemiology. However, some of the problems posed by this research will probably not be solved with the passage of time. The Russian National Medical and Dosimetric Registry contains estimates of exposure with associated errors that can be between 50% and 300%.[23] In January 2005 the database included individual medical and dosimetric data for 614,887 persons, including 186,395 liquidators and 367,850 residents of four contaminated *oblasts* of Western Russia.[24] These numbers contrast with the fact that liquidators were many more, possibly close to 800,000, many of them from non-Russian republics of the USSR, a multinational state now disappeared which, at the time of the Chernobyl disaster had 290 million inhabitants, most of which probably had some exposure to the radioactive fallout. Available dosimetric information looks dramatically insufficient. The war between Russia and Ukraine, launched by President

---

21 Hatch & Cardis (2017), "Somatic health effects of Chernobyl". Since presently CVD is the first cause of death in basically all countries, any increase, even small, in the mortaly from CVD has a major impact on total mortality.

22 Williams & Baverstock (2006), "The nuclear accident at Chernobyl exposed hundreds of thousands of people to radioactive fallout. We still have much to learn about its consequences", *Nature* 440, 993–994.

23 Pitkevitch et al. (1997), "Exposure levels for persons involved in recovery operations after the Chernobyl accident: Statistical analysis based on the data of the Russian National Medical and Dosimetric Registry", *Radiation & Environmental Biophysics* 36(3), 149–160.

24 Ivanov (2007), "Late cancer and noncancer risks among Chernobyl emergency workers of Russia", *Health Physics* 93(5), 470–479; Kashcheev et al. (2015), "Incidence and mortality of solid cancer among emergency workers of the Chernobyl accident: assessment of radiation risks for the follow-up period of 1992–2009", *Radiation & Environmental Biophysics* 54(1), 13–23.

Putin and still evolving at this writing, will probably make addressing these problems in the data even more difficult — if not impossible.

In 2006 the Chernobyl Forum basically rejected any effects of the Chernobyl fallout on health except the causation of thyroid cancers and a few thousand cases of other malignancies and basically dismissed the possibility of effects beyond Ukraine, Belarus, and Russia. In contrast to that limited view, research has produced strong evidence that the Chernobyl fallout is linked not only to cancer in children and adults, but also to effects ranging from disorders of the lung function in children[25] to CVD in adults.[26] This is consistent with other investigations showing probable causal associations between low-dose radiation and CVD.[27]

The most recent WHO evaluation of the consequences of Chernobyl reports health effects "in the three affected countries,"[28] including more than 11,000 childhood thyroid cancer cases that been diagnosed by 2016. The same source acknowledges emerging evidence — from studies of Chernobyl, of workers in the nuclear industry and of medically exposed populations — that low-dose protracted exposures to radiation increase the relative risk of cancer; and that suggestive evidence of increased risk of CVD linked to ionizing radiation has been supported both by Chernobyl investigations and by a meta-analysis of a variety of studies.

In the early years after Chernobyl, it was often mentioned by the experts of the IAEA and other specialized agencies that the main health impact of Chernobyl in the affected populations of Ukraine, Belarus and Russia has been the emergence of radiophobia, and irrational fear that would be the main reason for a number of disorders that in no way could be attributed to the low levels of radiation received by these populations. This claim has been proved wrong for many specific health outcomes, although it is undeniable that a number of health consequences of the nuclear disaster may have been mediated by psychological mechanisms linked to fear of exposure to intangible threats, fear for exposed children, mistrust of authorities or the stress of forced evacuations. All these factors may have led to psychological distress, dietary changes to avoid

---

25 Svendsen et al. (2010), "[137]Cesium exposure and spirometry measures in Ukrainian children affected by the Chernobyl nuclear incident", *Environmental Health Perspectives* 118(5), 720–725.
26 Samet et al. (2018), "Gilbert W. Beebe Symposium".
27 Little et al. (2012), "Systematic review and meta-analysis of circulatory disease from exposure to low-level ionizing radiation and estimates of potential population mortality risks", *Environmental Health Perspectives* 120(11), 1503–1511.
28 WHO (2016), "1986–2016: Chernobyl at 30: An update", accessed April 2020.

contamination, or consumption of alcohol, cigarettes or other drugs, so that a fraction of deaths from suicide, cirrhosis, or lung cancer "could be regarded as indirect consequences of the accident and the subsequent measures taken".[29]

A recent investigation of the long-term effects of the 1986 Chernobyl catastrophe in a nationally representative survey in Ukraine included some 6000 individuals who according to their places of residence had been exposed to low levels of radiation after the disaster in 1986. Large and persistent psychological effects of the nuclear disaster were found, with individuals who had been more exposed exhibiting poorer subjective well-being, higher depression rates and lower subjective survival probabilities.[30]

The view that the effects of Chernobyl are fundamentally limited to Ukraine, Belarus and Russia has been frequently sustained actively or passively by specialized agencies like IAEA, UNSCEAR and WHO, but evidence against this view has been steadily emerging over time. Early epidemiologic evidence gathered in the 1990s on the relation of Chernobyl fallout with the risk of leukemia in childhood in countries that had not been in the USSR produced inconclusive results[31] and it was evaluated quite differently by different authors[32] and even by the same authors after a longer follow-up period.[33] In 2006, a group which included many of the top researchers on epidemiological effects of radiation used the available evidence to estimate the expected cancer burden from radioactive fallout from Chernobyl in European countries that had not belonged to the USSR. They concluded that about 5,000 cancer cases (1,000 of them thyroid cancer) had already occurred by 2006, and that 41,000 additional cancer cases (in-

---

29 Baverstock & Williams (2006), The Chernobyl accident 20 years on: An assessment of the health consequences and the international response", *Environmental Health Perspectives* 114, 1312–1317.

30 Danzer & Danzer (2016), "The long-run consequences of Chernobyl: Evidence on subjective well-being, mental health and welfare", *Journal of Public Economics* 135, 47–60.

31 Moysich et al. (2002), "Chernobyl-related ionising radiation exposure and cancer risk: An epidemiological review", *Lancet Oncology* 3(5), 269–279; Ivanov (2007), "Late cancer and non-cancer risks"; Pitkevitch et al. (1997), "Exposure levels".

32 Hoffmann (2002), "Has fallout from the Chernobyl accident caused childhood leukaemia in Europe? A commentary on the epidemiologic evidence", *European Journal of Public Health* 12(1), 72–76; Cardis et al. (2006), "Cancer consequences of the Chernobyl accident: 20 years on", *Journal of Radiological Protection* 26(2), 127–140.

33 Petridou et al. (1994), "Trends and geographical distribution of childhood leukemia in Greece in relation to the Chernobyl accident", *Scandinavian Journal of Social Medicine* 22(2), 127–131; Petridou et al. (1997), "Infant leukaemia after in utero exposure to radiation from Chernobyl", *Nature* 387(6630), 246.

cluding 16,000 cases of thyroid cancer) would occur by 2065.[34] The 95% uncertainty interval for all Chernobyl-related cancers until 2065 was 14,400 to 131,000, a very large range. At any rate, with several hundred million cancer cases expected by 2065 from other causes, the authors concluded that it was unlikely that the cancer burden from Chernobyl could be detected in national cancer statistics. But the link between Chernobyl fallout and cancer in countries beyond the old USSR can also be investigated in other ways as shown by an important study on the effects of low-dose radiation from the Chernobyl fallout on the incidence of cancer, authored in 2018 by Francesca Marino and Luca Nunziata, two Italian economists. These researchers classified 80 regions belonging to 13 European countries — Austria, the Czech Republic, Denmark, Estonia, France, Germany, Ireland, Latvia, Lithuania, Luxembourg, Netherlands, Portugal, and Spain — into four levels of fallout deposition (none, low, medium, and high deposition) according to the cesium-137 fallout estimated to have been deposited by the Chernobyl disaster in 1986. Then they examined the hospital discharges after treatment for neoplasms in these regions in the period 2000 – 2013. The overall population average was around 1.7 hospital discharges per 100 inhabitants, but discharges were, respectively, 0.36, 0.44, and 0.98 per 100 inhabitants higher in the regions of low, medium, and high deposition compared to regions with no deposition of cesium-137. The result was robust to different model specifications and tests and the authors concluded that radioactive fallout is positively associated with a higher incidence of hospital discharges after treatment for neoplasms almost 30 years after its release, with larger effects in regions where the radioactivity was more intense. They also concluded that their estimates were comparable to the findings of studies on the long-term health effects of continuous low levels of radiation exposure among workers in the nuclear industry.[35]

The notion that the observable effects of the Chernobyl nuclear disaster were restricted to just three Republics of the old USSR looks quite clearly proved to be wrong.

---

34 Cardis et al. (2006), "Estimates of the cancer burden in Europe from radioactive fallout from the Chernobyl accident", *International Journal of Cancer* 119(6), 1224 – 1235.
35 Marino & Nunziata (2018), "Long-term consequences of the Chernobyl radioactive fallout: An exploration of the aggregate data", *Milbank Quarterly* 96(4), 814 – 857.

Chapter 12
Mortality effects of fallout from nuclear tests

As explained in chapter 7, in the 1950s and early 1960s almost 200 nuclear explosions took place in the atmosphere at the Nuclear Test Site in southern Nevada. Despite claims by the AEC that the tests had no effects beyond the testing ground and did not raise radioactivity above safe levels, evidence to the contrary was soon noticed by residents in Nevada, Arizona and Utah who had not been given any instruction to protect themselves. Despite reassurance by government officials that there was no risk, not only a few thousand sheep died but symptoms such as nausea, headaches, burns and blisters on the exposed skin, and hair loss were noticed by the ranchers and other residents in the downwind areas. In the following years many children developed leukemia and cancers rates evidently rose in the downwind areas. Litigation developed resulting into judicial decisions that were most frequently favorable to the government. However, with the passage of time, it became increasingly evident that many cancer deaths could be linked to the fallout from the Nevada tests, and that the US government had been deceiving its own citizens for years. It is a long and sad story that has been told in many books and articles.[1] In a study published in 1990 in which cases of acute leukemia in the fallout area were compared with controls, a clear association was found between leukemias discovered from 1952 to 1963 and the external radiation dose from the fallout received by the bone marrow of individuals who were younger than 20 years at exposure.[2]

Increasing evidence is emerging however that the consequences of nuclear tests go beyond extra cases of leukemia, thyroid cancer, and other malignancies. A recent paper by a group of Norwegian authors led by Sandra E. Black examined the association of levels of radiation exposure in utero resulting from nuclear weapon testing in the 1950s and early 1960s with the long-tem outcomes of Norwegian children. Low-dose radiation, specifically during months 3 and 4 in utero, was found leading to lower IQ scores for men and lower education attainment and earnings among men and women. The authors concluded that given the lack of awareness about nuclear testing in Norway during the 1950s and

---

1 Fradkin (1989), *Fallout — An American nuclear tragedy*; Udal (1994), *The myths of August*; Lifton & Mitchell (1995), *Hiroshima in America: Fifty years of denial*; Ball (1986), "Downwind from the bomb", *The New York Times Magazine* Feb. 9, 33; Brodie (2015), "Radiation secrecy and censorship after Hiroshima and Nagasaki", *Journal of Social History* 48(4), 842–864.
2 Stevens et al. (1990), "Leukemia in Utah and radioactive fallout from the Nevada test site: A case-control study", *JAMA* 94, 585–591.

https://doi.org/10.1515/9783110761788-016

1960s, their estimates are very unlikely to be affected by avoidance behavior or stress effects, so they are very likely causal effects.[3]

In recent years several investigations have indicated that the number of deaths caused by the fallout from nuclear tests in the US population very likely is in the order of hundreds of thousands. In 2006, researchers from the National Cancer Institute evaluated the effect of the fallout from nuclear tests in Nevada on the incidence of thyroid cancer in the US considering the radiation levels in different areas and the known carcinogenic effects of the radioisotopes deposited. They estimated that about 49,000 fallout-related cases might occur in the US, almost all of them among persons who were under age 20 at some time during the period 1951–1957. The 95% confidence interval for this number of cancers was 11,300 to 212,000, and accounting for the extra thyroid exposure due to global fallout, the estimated excess would increase by 10%, from 49,000 to 54,000. In the same investigation it was estimated that about 22,000 radiation-related cancers, half of them fatal, might result from the external exposure of the US population to the fallout from nuclear tests.[4]

Keith Meyers, an economist at the University of Southern Denmark, has investigated links between the deposition from fallout of the nuclear tests that were performed in Nevada in the 1950s and agricultural output, cancer mortality, and all-cause mortality registered in subsequent years in the counties of the continental US. Meyers has shown that the radioactive fallout from nuclear tests had an adverse significant effect on the agricultural production of the central areas of the US.[5] This by itself would show that the economic and environmental impact of nuclear testing goes much beyond than previously thought. Even states as far from Nevada as Maine were exposed to radioactive iodine through milk in the days after tests. Using data from close to 3000 counties of the continental US, Meyers has shown also that the fallout deposition from these nuclear tests has a statistically significant effect on county mortality rates. In a paper still unpublished, considering the period starting in 1951, Meyers finds a consistent relationship between fallout in the countries of the US from the tests in Nevada and both cancer mortality and all-cause mortality in these counties. He shows that the arrival of fallout resulted in a sharp increase in mortality for at least ten years. His main results suggest that the nuclear tests in Nevada contributed to approxi-

3 Black et al. (2019), "This is only a test? Long-run and intergenerational impacts of prenatal exposure to radioactive fallout", *Review of Economics and Statistics* 101 (3), 531–546.
4 Simon et al. (2006), "Fallout from nuclear weapons tests and cancer risks", *American Scientist* 94(1), 48–57.
5 Meyers (2019). In the shadow of the mushroom cloud: Nuclear testing, radioactive fallout, and damage to US Agriculture, 1945 to 1970", *Journal of Economic History* 79(1), 244–274.

mately 360,000 deaths from all causes and 81,000 cancer deaths.[6] The estimates of Meyers appear sound and they are consistent with investigations that have shown effects of low dose radiation not only on cancer rates but also on CVD mortality rates after exposure to low doses of radiation.[7]

According to expert testimony before the US Senate, the amount of radioactivity from radioactive iodine released by the Chernobyl disaster was about 45 million curies, compared to 145 million curies released from the atmospheric detonations of nuclear bombs in Nevada.[8] But the nuclear tests in Nevada were only a portion of the 2056 atomic tests that have been performed to date, of which 528 were atmospheric tests realized in different parts of our planet including the Southwest US, the Pacific Ocean, the Artic, Kazakhstan, Uzbekistan, Ukraine, Argelia, Australia, Eastern China and probably the Indian Ocean.[9] As Kate Brown has argued, Chernobyl was the disaster that, if examined too closely, could open the Pandora's box of lawsuits against multiple governments that tested hundreds of atomic bombs openly in the atmosphere.[10]

In the US both incidence and mortality of thyroid cancer are increasing,[11] and similar trends are reported in other countries, and globally.[12] WHO has stated that in evaluating the consequences of Chernobyl it should be noted that a general increase in cancer incidence has been reported in recent decades worldwide.[13] Of course, there can be many reasons for a worldwide increase in the incidence of cancer, including perhaps earlier and more frequent detection of tumors that in less medicalized times would mostly go undetected. However, the increasing level of ionizing radiation from multiple sources — including Chernobyl, tests of atomic weapons, accidents and normal working of nuclear plants, medical uses, etc. — is also consistent with that trend.

---

6 Meyers (2022), "Some unintended fallout from defense policy: Measuring the effect of atmospheric nuclear testing on American mortality patterns".
7 National Research Council (2006), *Health risks from exposure to low levels of ionizing radiation: BEIR VII Phase 2*, 160, 185 – 187; Hatch & Cardis (2017), "Somatic health effects of Chernobyl".
8 Brown (2019), *Manual for survival — A Chernobyl guide to the future*, 246.
9 Arms Control Association, "The Nuclear Testing Tally", accessed February 2022.
10 Brown (2019), *Manual for survival*, 5.
11 Lim et al. (2017), "Trends in thyroid cancer incidence and mortality in the United States, 1974 – 2013", *JAMA* 317(13), 1338 – 1348.
12 Deng et al. (2020), "Global burden of thyroid cancer from 1990 to 2017", *JAMA Network Open* 3(6), e208759- e208759; Ivanova et al. (2020), "Thyroid cancer incidence in Bulgaria before and after the introduction of universal salt iodization", *Balkan Medical Journal* 37(6), 330 – 335.
13 WHO (2016), "1986 – 2016: Chernobyl at 30 – An update."

Unfortunately, the health implications of Chernobyl have been obfuscated and their recognition (or lack of recognition) impacted by the stance of governments and other players on nuclear power and by political considerations. Knowledgeable observers have asserted that a resolute attempt to "close the Chernobyl book" occurred in 2006, with some UN agencies strongly agreeing. Political interference has resulted in unwillingness to seek the truth.[14]

The evidence of the harmful effects of radioactivity on health has accumulated in the past two decades, despite powerful attempts to minimize the risks of low-dose radiation generated by atomic tests, mining and manufacturing of radioactive substances, nuclear power plants, medical uses of radioisotopes, and other sources. The glamour that nuclear energy had in the first half of the past century has yielded in the present century to a fear that is to a large extent based in fact. The reality is that even when the monster appeared to be domesticated and atomic energy was harnessed for peaceful purposes, it generated very serious unintended consequences. Chernobyl has been a major chapter in that story.

---

14 Baverstock (2011), "Chernobyl 25 years on", *BMJ* 342, d2443.

Chapter 13
Conclusion

The transitional mortality crisis that was suffered by the countries of the old Soviet bloc was the longest in Ukraine, Belarus, Russia, and Bulgaria. Measured by the period of reduced life expectancy for males, which indicates increased levels of mortality, the mortality crisis lasted 29 years in Ukraine, 28 in Belarus, 26 in Russia, and 22 in Bulgaria (see Tabs 1.1 and 1.2 and Figs. 1.1 and 1.2 on pages 2 and 4). There is consensus that Ukraine, Belarus, and Russia were the three countries that suffered the worst radioactive fallout from the Chernobyl disaster, while data on radioactive fallout in Bulgaria are remarkably absent except by unofficial reports that claim levels of radioactivity hundreds of times higher than former background levels in the spring of 1986, after a heavy radioactive fallout in the days following the Chernobyl disaster. Thus it seems reasonable to assume that Ukraine, Belarus, Russia, and Bulgaria are the four countries of the old Soviet bloc that were the most contaminated by the fallout from the Chernobyl disaster and notably they were also the four countries in which the mortality crisis that started in the late 1980s lasted the most.

Significant changes in life expectancy trends emerged around the time of the Chernobyl disaster. In Belarus and Ukraine, the life expectancy (LEB) of males peaked in 1986, in Russia in 1987, which means that mortality started to increase immediately after the Chernobyl disaster, several years before the Soviet Union crashed and ex-Soviet citizens were suddenly exposed to all kinds of adversities that undoubtedly increased mortality. In Bulgaria male LEB had a peak of 68.7 years in 1986, the year of the Chernobyl disaster, and then decreased to 68.4 in 1987, to stagnate and drop steadily during the 1990s reaching a low of 67.0 in 1997. It was not until the year 2004 that male LEB reached 69.1 years in Bulgaria, the first time after Chernobyl that LEB was higher than pretransitional levels (Table C-1 in Appendix C).

The evolution of birth rates in these four countries is also consistent with an effect of the Chernobyl disaster. Indeed, in Russia, Ukraine, and Belarus the birth rate started to decline quickly immediately after 1986, despite the fact that had been oscillating without a clear trend since 1968 (see Fig. 4.1, page 34). In Bulgaria birth rates were already showing a clear declining trend before 1986, but overall, the evolution of the birth rate in that country does not look inconsistent with an effect of the Chernobyl disaster.

The evolution of LEB and birth rates in the Baltic nations, Estonia, Latvia, and Lithuania (Fig. 1.3, page 5, Fig. 4.2, page 35) is also consistent with an effect of the Chernobyl disaster: in these three countries both LEB and birth rates

https://doi.org/10.1515/9783110761788-017

showed changes in trends right after the Chernobyl disaster. LEB which had been rising since 1980, started declining in 1987 in Lithuania, in 1988 in Latvia, and in 1989 in Estonia. Birth rates peaked in 1986 in Lithuania and Latvia and in 1987 in Estonia, then declined quickly. As it was explained in chapter 4, changes in sex ratios at birth after 1986 in Eastern Europe and the countries of the old USSR are also consistent with a radiobiological effect on fetuses and germ cells of the radioactive fallout from the Chernobyl disaster.

These "coincidental" changes in trends of demographic indicators closely aligned with the time of the Chernobyl disaster have been rarely noticed. Many things occurred in the countries of the old USSR and Eastern Europe and could explain these trends. The Chernobyl disaster is certainly one of them.

In the 1950s atomic energy was promoted as the technological development that would open the door to an era of abundance. Nuclear reactors in each household would generate cheap electricity and hot water; airplanes would fly powered by atomic energy; atomic explosives would be used like dynamite to open channels and remove obstacles for public infrastructures; different types of radiation would be major tools for diagnostic or therapeutic medical purposes. Most of these things turned out to be just fantasies, but at the time X-rays were used happily to examine pregnant women or fit shoes to children, and until the 1970s or the 1980s radiation was often used as therapy for innocuous ailments. As discussed in this book, over the past two decades evidence of the harmful effects of low-dose exposure to ionizing radiation has accumulated. Dozens of investigations of the long-term effects of acute exposure to ionizing radiation in the survivors of the bombings of Hiroshima and Nagasaki, of chronic exposures in uranium miners and workers of the nuclear industries, of exposures to medical uses of radiation in patients, and of populations exposed to the fallout of nuclear tests or nuclear disasters, have shown that radiation is causally connected to many forms of cancer but also to other ailments like CVD, which is the first cause of death in modern societies. In addition, many early views on the biological effects of radiation based on the initial analyses of Japanese survivors of the 1945 atomic bombings have been challenged by subsequent follow-up studies of these survivors, as well as by recent investigations of nuclear workers, populations exposed to the fallout of the Chernobyl disaster, medical X-rays, and other sources of ionizing radiation.[1] Therefore, there is ample basis on which to hypothesize and investigate to what extent the Cherno-

---

1 Gayle Greene has written very eloquently on all this in her biographical contributions on Alice Stewart: Greene (2011), "Richard Doll and Alice Stewart: Reputation and the shaping of scientific 'truth'", *Perspectives in Biology & Medicine* 54(4), 504–531; Greene (2017), *The woman who knew too much: Alice Stewart and the secrets of radiation*.

byl disaster may have contributed to the significant mortality crisis experienced between the late 1980s and the early years of the 21st century by the countries of Eastern Europe and the old USSR, one of the most important health disasters of the modern era. Unfortunately, present war conditions in Ukraine will not be favorable at all to the development of such investigations.

Atomic energy is still seen by some scientists and governments as the key to avoiding catastrophic climate change or to reducing dependency on foreign energy sources.[2] Certainly, the production of electricity using nuclear plants is somewhat "clean" in the sense of not generating emissions of greenhouse gases (though even existing plants imply some emissions due to the need for continuous mining and refining of uranium, and the water vapor and heat they release). However, nuclear power can have unintended adverse consequences, as discussed in this book, and it is neither renewable nor cheap and does not lead to energy independence.

If a nuclear war does not eliminate all the problems of humanity by eliminating humanity itself or by sending surviving humans back into caves, human civilization will face significant problems as we transition away from fossil fuels. Based on current knowledge and the lessons of history, including the lessons of Chernobyl, it seems doubtful that nuclear energy can help us produce a better future. There are better ways, the key issue is whether we will find them in time.[3]

---

2 A very illustrative example of the controversies on the use of atomic energy to prevent catastrophic climate change is the exchange between four prominent climate change scientists, including James Hansen (see the letter reproduced in Revkin, 2013) and four Japanese scholars, including Japan's former lead climate-treaty negotiator (Asuka et al. 2014). Both the Biden administration and the British government seem at the time of this writing ready to bid for nuclear energy; see Clifford (2022), "Why the U.S. government plans to spend billions to keep money-losing nuclear plants open", and Hunnicutt & Scheyderand (2022), "U.S. ban on Russian energy imports does not include uranium".

3 See Jacobson (2021b), "The 7 reasons why nuclear energy is not the answer to solve climate change", a summary of Jacobson (2021a), *100% Clean, Renewable Energy and Storage for Everything*.

Appendix A
Units for measurement of ionizing radiation

The *rad,* from *r*adiation *a*bsorbed *d*ose, was historically the standard unit of absorbed dose, equal to 100 ergs per gram.

The *gray* (symbol: Gy) is a unit of absorbed radiation defined as the absorption of one joule of radiation energy per kilogram of matter. The gray replaced the rad, with the equivalency 1 Gy = 100 rad.

The *roentgen,* also spelled *röntgen,* is a unit of exposure to *X*-rays or gamma radiation such that the charged particles liberated by the radiation reach a given amount of electric charge (2.58×10^{-4} coulomb per kilogram of air).

The *rem* (from *r*oentgen *e*quivalent *m*an) is a unit of ionizing radiation equal to the amount that produces the same damage to humans as 1 roentgen of high-voltage *X*-rays.

The *sievert* (symbol: Sv) is a unit of radiation dose, equal to 100 rem.

For practical purposes an exposure measured in roentgens can be considered equivalent to an absorbed dose measured in rads and equivalent to a dose equivalent measured in rems, as 1 roentgen and 1 rad are roughly equivalent in the case of beta or gamma radiation.

Often smaller units such as the millisievert (1 mSv = 0.001 Sv) or the millirem (1 mr = 0.001 r) are used. Making complicated things even more confusing, r is often used as the abbreviation of rad, rem or roentgen, but R is also sometimes used.

Sources: Knoll (2010), *Radiation detection and measurement*; Parker (1984), *McGraw-Hill dictionary of physics.*

https://doi.org/10.1515/9783110761788-018

Appendix B
Gender issues

I use life expectancy at birth (LEB) for males in most of the analyses of this book because there is no doubt that the mortality crisis in Eastern Europe and the USSR affected males much more than females. Since LEB for a given year is a kind of inverse quantifier of all the age-specific mortality rates observed that year, male LEB is a very precise index of the mortality that males suffered that year at all ages. Thus, to gauge the importance of the mortality crisis in Eastern Europe, male LEB looks a much better instrument than female LEB. Fig. B.1 and table B.1 in this appendix, correspond respectively to Table 1.1 and Fig. 1.2 of chapter 1, but these are elaborated with data for female LEB. Comparing Fig. 1.2 and Fig. B.1 it is easy to note the shape of the curves is not very different (for instance, the changes in trend around 1986 are present in graphs of both male and female LEB), but the oscillations are milder in the female LEB graphs and judging by the length and deepness of the mortality crisis for each country, as indicated by LEB, it is quite obvious that the crisis affected males much more severely.

An issue connected with this is whether radiation in general or the fallout from Chernobyl in particular affects more harmfully to males or to females. For instance, the induction of myeloid leukemia has been extensively studied in the CBA and RFM strains of mice, in which the susceptibility of female mice was found markedly lower.[1] In a study published in 1997, Delongchamp et al. analyzed data on cancer mortality among atomic bomb survivors who were exposed either in utero or during the first 5 years of life.[2] These included 807 individuals who had radiation exposure (at least 0.01 Sv) in utero and 5,545 persons who had had a similar exposure during childhood. The comparison group included 10,453 persons with very low (<0.01 Sv) or no exposure. Ten cancer deaths were observed in the cohort exposed in utero (1621 males and 1668 females), and a significant dose-response was observed with an estimated ERR/Sv (excess relative risk per sievert) of 2.1, with a 90% confidence interval of 0.2 to 6.0. An unusual aspect of the finding was that 9 of the 10 cancer deaths occurred in women, and significant differences between the men and women persisted when the three female cancer sites (breast, ovary, and uterus)

---

1 National Research Council (2006), *Health risks from exposure to low levels of ionizing radiation: BEIR VII Phase 2*, 73.

2 Delongchamp et al. (1997), "Cancer mortality among atomic bomb survivors exposed In utero or as young children, October 1950-May 1992", *Radiation Research* 147(3), 385–395.

https://doi.org/10.1515/9783110761788-019

were excluded from the analysis. Analyzing jointly the results in the cohorts exposed in utero or as young children, Delongchamp et al. concluded that in their results "women have a higher risk of mortality from solid cancer after radiation exposure than men" but commented that their results were based in a very small number of cancer deaths and should be interpreted with caution. The BEIR VII committee commented the findings in the paper by Delongchamp et al. stating that, in the medical literature on cancerogenic effects of radiation, minimal information exists "with respect to sex-specific effects, and none reports a gender-specific association between radiation and cancer."[3]

As explained in chapter 11, emerging evidence suggests that low-dose radiation increases the risk of CVD, but in the case of Chernobyl that evidence is derived from studies in liquidators who were almost 100% males. To my knowledge, there is no evidence suggesting a differential risk by gender of developing CVD as an effect of exposure to radiation. Evidence that ionizing radiation increases the proportion of males at birth by mechanisms still not well known seems to be solid though disputed.[4]

Some reasons suggest, I believe, that in the specific case of the Chernobyl fallout, males may have been more exposed to radiation than females. Not only because the close-to-a million liquidators were mostly males, but also because men tend to stay outdoors more time than women and if that is the case, overall radiation exposure will be greater because it is outdoor where the radioactive materials like cesium-137 or other radionuclides dropped after the explosions and fires in the reactor number 4 of the nuclear power plant of Chernobyl.

---

3 National Research Council (2006), *Health risks from exposure*, 151, 330.
4 See the exchange between Scherb & Voigt (2011 and 2012) and Bochud & Jung (2011).

Tab. B1: Length and deepness of the mortality crisis in the fifteen republics of the former USSR as assessed from the year and value of the pre-crisis peak in life expectancy for females (LEBf), the year and value of the next trough in LEBf, and the year in which the pre-crisis peak was surpassed.

	A	B	C	D	E	F = E-A	G = D-B
	Peak		Trough				
Country	Year	LEBf	Year	LEBf	Recovery	Length	Deepness
Georgia	1991	76.7	2003	74.7	1995	4	2.0
Tajikistan	1991	72.7	1993	68.2	1997	6	4.6
Azerbaijan	1990	75.3	1994	73.1	1998	8	2.2
Lithuania	1989	76.4	1994	74.9	1997	8	1.5
Estonia	1987	75.0	1994	73.0	1996	9	2.0
Turkmenistan	1990	70.0	1994	66.6	1999	9	3.4
Latvia	1989	75.2	1994	72.6	1999	10	2.6
Kyrgyzstan	1990	73.0	1994	69.9	2001	11	3.1
Uzbekistan	1990	72.9	1994	70.2	2004	14	2.7
Moldova	1989	72.3	1995	69.7	2004	15	2.6
Armenia	1981	76.9	1993	74.6	1998	17	2.2
Belarus	1989	76.4	1996	73.9	2008	19	2.5
Kazakhstan	1990	73.4	1996	70.3	2009	19	3.1
Russia	1989	74.6	1994	71.2	2009	20	3.4
Ukraine	1989	75.3	1995	72.6	2011	22	2.7

Author's elaboration from data in the WHO-HFA database.

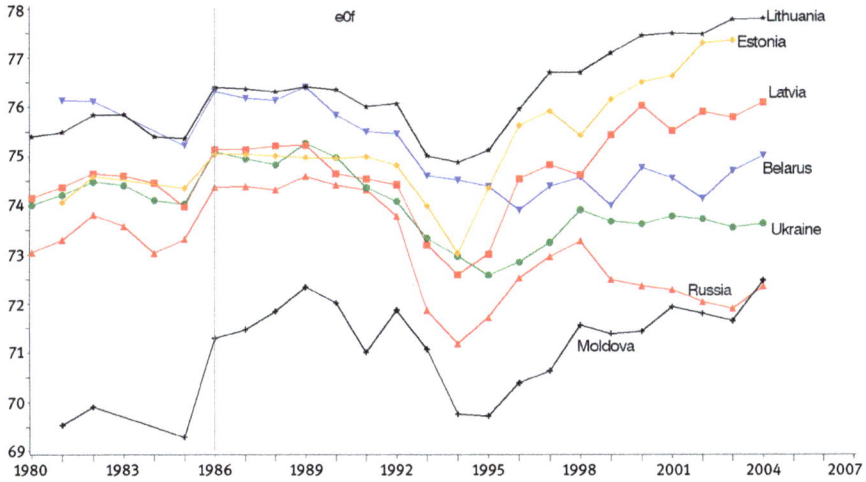

Fig. B1: Life expectancy at birth for females in the Western republics of the former USSR, 1980 – 2004. The vertical line marks 1986, the year in which the Chernobyl disaster occurred. Author's elaboration from data in the HFA database, WHO-Europe.

Appendix C
Data Tables

https://doi.org/10.1515/9783110761788-020

Tab. C1: Life expectancy at birth for males, republics of the USSR, before and after the breakdown of the USSR in 1991

Year	RUS	BLR	UKR	LVA	EST	LTU	MDA	AZE	GEO	ARM	KAZ	KGZ	TJK	TKM	UZB
1980	61.4		64.6	63.8		65.4				69.6		61.2			63.6
1981	61.7	66	64.7	63.4	64.0	65.3	62.7	64.9	67.0	70.4	61.5	62.2	64.5	60.0	64.7
1982	62.4	66.3	64.9	64.3	64.4	65.7	63.0	65.7	67.6	70.1	61.9	63.0	64.6	61.2	63.9
1983	62.3		64.9	63.9		65.9				69.8		62.9			63.9
1984	61.7		64.6	64.1		65.2				69.4		62.0			63.7
1985	62.8	66.1	65.2	64.7	64.6	65.6	62.8	66.0	67.8	69.9	62.6	63.0	66.4	61.2	64.8
1986	64.9	67.8	67.0	66.3	66.2	67.8	65.0	66.4	67.9	70.4	64.2	65.4	67.0	61.1	65.5
1987	64.9	67.6	66.7	66.4	66.3	67.7	65.6	66.5	68.2	70.5	64.2	64.7	66.8	62.1	65.7
1988	64.7	67.3	66.6	66.3	66.5	67.5	65.4	65.9	68.0	60.7	64.0	64.3	66.0	61.9	65.5
1989	64.2	66.8	66.2	65.4	65.8	66.9	65.6	66.8	68.2	69.2	63.9	64.3	66.9	61.9	66.1
1990	63.8	66.3	65.7	64.3	64.7	66.5	65.0	67.1	69.1	68.6	63.9	64.4	67.1	63.0	66.3
1991	63.5	65.6	64.7	63.7	64.4	65.2	64.2	66.6	69.0	69.1	63.4	64.6	67.4	62.2	65.8
1992	62.1	65.1	63.9	62.7	63.5	64.9	63.9	64.1	68.8	67.9	63.3	64.2	65.2	62.6	65.6
1993	58.9	63.8	63.2	60.5	62.4	63.1	64.1	63.9		67.6	61.2	62.5	56.4	61.4	65.1
1994	57.7	63.5	62.5	59.2	60.8	62.6	62.3	62.9	70.0	68.6	60.8	61.1	63.2	61.6	64.7
1995	58.4	62.9	61.3	60.2	61.5	63.3	62.0	65.4	71.0	69.7	59.3	61.3	65.5	62.1	65.0
1996	59.8	63.4	61.7	63.0	64.3	64.7	63.0	66.4	70.5	70.1	58.9	62.5	65.9	61.5	65.0
1997	61.1	62.9	62.4	63.9	64.4	65.5	63.2	67.0	69.8	71.3	59.4	62.5	67.6	62.2	66.0
1998	61.4	62.7	63.3	63.5	64.1	66.0	64.2	67.9	69.8	72.5	59.4	63.2	68.8	62.5	66.1
1999	60	62.3	62.8	64.8	65.0	66.4	63.8	68.1	70.0	72.6	60.8	64.5	69.9	64.1	67.2
2000	59.2	63.4	62.3	64.8	65.9	66.8	64.0	68.7	70.4	73.5	60.2	63.8	70.7	64.3	67.0
2001	59.1	62.8	62.6	64.3	65.4	65.9	64.5	69.7	70.9	73.7	60.6	64.6	70.3	65.8	67.6
2002	59	62.3	62.2	64.5	65.7	66.2	64.4	69.8	68.0	69.9	61.0	64.1	70.3	65.5	67.6
2003	58.7	62.7	62.3	65.4	66.5	66.4	64.4	69.5	69.1	70.0	60.7	64.1	70.7	65.5	68.0
2004	59.1	63.2	62.0	65.6	66.8	66.3	64.6	69.9	68.0		60.8	64.2	71.1	66.3	68.8
2005	59.1	62.9	61.5	65.0	67.6	65.2	63.8		70.1		60.4	63.9	71.2	65.4	68.1

Tab. C1: Life expectancy at birth for males, republics of the USSR, before and after the breakdown of the USSR in 1991 *(Continued)*

Year	RUS	BLR	UKR	LVA	EST	LTU	MDA	AZE	GEO	ARM	KAZ	KGZ	TJK	TKM	UZB
2006	60.5		62.3	65.0	67.7	65.1	64.6		70.0		60.7	63.5		66.2	
2007	61.6	64.6	61.8	65.3	67.6	64.5	65.2	71.3	70.6		60.8	63.8		66.3	
2008	62	64.7	62.3	66.5	69.0	66.0	65.5			70.4	62.0	64.6		66.8	
2009	62.9	64.8	64.4	67.5	70.0	67.2	65.3		69.3	70.6	63.7	65.1		68.0	70.7
2010	63.2	64.6	65.2	67.9	70.9	67.6	64.9		70.3		63.7	65.5		67.8	70.7
2011	64.2	64.8	66.0	68.6	71.5	68.1	66.8		70.3		64.4	66.0		67.9	70.7
2012	64.7		66.2	68.9	71.5	68.5	67.2		70.4	71.3	65.0	66.3		68.3	70.7
2013	65.3	67.3		69.4	72.6	68.6	68.2		71.0	72.0	66.0	67.0		67.3	71.2
2014		67.9	66.3	69.5	72.4	69.2	67.6		68.8	71.8	67.1	67.1			71.2
2015			67.5	70.1	73.3	69.2	67.6		68.7	71.8	67.5	68.0			
2016						69.5	68.2								

Data from the HFA database of the European Office of WHO, accessed September 2019. Empty cells correspond to data unreported in the HFA database. RUS, Russia; BLR, Belarus; UKR, Ukraine; LVA, Latvia; EST, Estonia; LTU, Lithuania; MDA, Moldova; AZE, Azerbaijan; GEO, Georgia; ARM, Armenia, KAZ, Kazakhstan; KGZ, Kyrgyzstan; TJK, Tajikistan; TKM, Turkmenistan, UZB, Uzbekistan.

Tab. C2: Life expectancy at birth for males in the countries of Eastern Europe and the Balkans that were centrally planned economies, before and after the transition to a market economy around 1990

Year	ALB	BGR	BIH	CZE	DEU	HRV	MKD	MNE	POL	HUN	ROU	SRB	SVK	SVN
1980		68.5		66.8						65.5	66.6		66.8	
1981		69.0		67.2						65.5	66.8			
1982		68.5		67.3						65.7	67.1		67.0	
1983		68.5		67.0						65.1	67.0			
1984		68.5		67.3						65.1	67.1		66.8	
1985		68.4	68.6			67.6		72.3	66.5	65.2	66.5		66.9	68.0
1986		68.7	69.1	67.6		68.0		72.7	66.7	65.4	66.8		67.0	68.6
1987	69.5	68.4	69.2	67.9		67.9		73.8	66.8	65.7	66.2		68.0	68.3
1988	69.8	68.3	69.2	68.1		68.0		74.9	67.1	66.2	66.5		67.5	69.0
1989	69.2	68.3	69.4	68.2		68.6		74.4	66.8	65.5	66.7		67.0	69.4
1990	69.6	68.3	70.1	67.6	72.1	68.7		74.3	66.6	65.2	66.6		66.8	70.0
1991		68.4	69.5	68.3	72.2	66.1	69.9	71.8	66.2	65.2	66.9		66.9	69.6
1992	69.8	67.8		68.6	72.7	67.1	69.0	71.0	66.7	64.7	66.1		67.7	69.7
1993	70.3	67.6		69.3	72.8	68.5	69.5	72.1	67.4	64.6	65.9		68.4	69.4
1994	72.1	67.2		69.5	73.1	69.2	69.8	72.2	67.5	65.0	65.7		68.4	70.2
1995	71.7	67.4		69.8	73.4	69.3	70.0	71.9	67.7	65.5	65.5		68.4	70.9
1996	71.4	67.5		70.5	73.7	68.7	70.5	71.7	68.2	66.3	65.1		68.9	71.2
1997	71.1	67.0		70.6	74.2	68.7	70.5	71.1	68.5	66.7	65.3		68.9	71.2
1998	71.7	67.4		71.2	74.6	68.6	70.4		68.9	66.5	66.3	69.1	68.6	71.3
1999	73.0	68.4		71.5	74.9	68.9	70.5		68.9	66.4	67.1	69.1	69.1	71.8
2000	72.2	68.5		71.7	75.2	69.1	71.1	71.5	69.6	67.2	67.8	69.0	69.3	72.3
2001	74.1	68.5		72.2	75.7	71.0	71.1	71.5	70.0	68.3	67.7	69.7	69.6	72.3
2002	73.8	68.9		72.2	75.8	71.2	70.8	71.6	70.4	68.4	67.4	69.8	69.9	72.7
2003	73.3	69.0		72.1	75.9	71.2	71.1	71.6	70.5	68.4	67.7	70.0	69.9	72.6
2004	73.7	69.1		72.6	76.6	72.1	71.6	71.6	70.7	68.8	68.3	70.1	70.4	73.6

Tab. C2: Life expectancy at birth for males in the countries of Eastern Europe and the Balkans that were centrally planned economies, before and after the transition to a market economy around 1990 (*Continued*)

Year	ALB	BGR	BIH	CZE	DEU	HRV	MKD	MNE	POL	HUN	ROU	SRB	SVK	SVN
2005	74.4	69.1		73.0	76.8	71.9	71.7	71.4	70.8	68.7	68.8	70.2	70.3	74.0
2006	75.4	69.3		73.5	77.3	72.6	71.8	71.6	71.0	69.2	69.2	70.8	70.5	74.5
2007	77.2	69.6		73.8	77.5	72.4	71.8	72.2	71.0	69.4	69.7	71.0	70.7	74.8
2008	76.4	69.8		74.2	77.7	72.5	72.5	72.8	71.3	70.0	69.8	71.4	70.9	75.7
2009	77.5	70.2		74.3	77.9	73.0	72.4	73.3	71.6	70.3	69.9	71.4	71.5	76.0
2010		70.3		74.6	78.1	73.6	73.0		72.3	70.8	70.2	71.8	71.8	76.6
2011		70.7	74.2	74.9	78.5	74.0	73.2		72.6	71.3	71.0	72.1		76.9
2012		71.0		75.1	78.7	74.0	73.1		72.7	71.6	71.0	72.4	72.6	77.2
2013		71.4		75.3	78.2	74.5	73.5		73.1	72.2	71.5	72.7	73.0	77.3
2014		71.1	75.2	75.9	78.8	74.8			73.8	72.4	71.5	72.9	73.4	78.3
2015				75.8	78.4	74.4			73.6	72.4	71.6	72.8		77.9
2016						75.0				72.7	71.8			

Data from the HFA database of the European Office of WHO. Empty cells are unreported data in the HFA database. ALB, Albania; BGR. Bulgaria; BIH, Bosnia and Herzegovina; CZE, Czech Republic; DEU, East Germany; HRV, Croatia; MKD, North Macedonia; MNE, Montenegro; POL, Poland; HUN, Hungary; ROU, Rumania; SRB, Serbia, SVK, Slovakia; SVN, Slovenia.

References

Ad hoc Working Group, US Department of Health & Human Services, Public Health Service, NIH. (1985). *Report of the NIH ad hoc working group to develop radioepidemiological tables – NIH publication no. 85–2748.* Washington, DC: US Government Printing Office.

Alexievich, S. (2017). *Second-hand time* (B. Shayevich Trans.). New York: Random House.

Alexievich, S. (2019). *Voices from Chernobyl: The oral history of a nuclear disaster* (K. Gessen Trans.). Champaign, IL: Dalkey Archive Press.

Alinaghizadeh, H., Tondel, M., & Walinder, R. (2014). Cancer incidence in northern Sweden before and after the Chernobyl nuclear power plant accident. *Radiation & Environmental Biophysics, 53*, 495–504.

Alinaghizadeh, H., Wålinder, R., Vingård, E., & Tondel, M. (2016). Total cancer incidence in relation to ^{137}Cs fallout in the most contaminated counties in sweden after the Chernobyl nuclear power plant accident: A register-based study. *BMJ Open, 6*(12), e011924.

Almond, D., Edlund, L., & Palme, M. (2009). Chernobyl's subclinical legacy: Prenatal exposure to radioactive fallout and school outcomes in sweden. *Quarterly Journal of Economics 124*(4), 1729–1772.

Altman, D. G., & Bland, J. M. (1995). Absence of evidence is not evidence of absence. *BMJ 326*(7401), 1267.

Andreev, E., Bogoyavlensky, D., & Stickley, A. (2013). Comparing alcohol mortality in tsarist and contemporary russia: Is the current situation historically unique? *Alcohol and Alcoholism 48*(2), 215–221.

Anonymous (2009). Ex-communist reform: Mass murder and the market. *The Economist,* Jan 22.

Archer, V. E. (1977). Occupational exposure to radiation as a cancer hazard. *Cancer 34* (4 Supp), 1802–1806.

Arms Control Association.The nuclear testing tally. Retrieved March 2022 from www.armscontrol.org/factsheets/nucleartesttally

Asuka, J., Park, S., Nishimura, M. & Morotomi, T. (2014). Reply to the letter from Dr. Hansen and others: Nuclear power is not the answer to climate change mitigation. Retrieved April 2022 from www.cneas.tohoku.ac.jp/labs/china/asuka/_src/2014/nuclear_power-climate_change_enver2.pdf

Axelrod, D., Burns, K., Davis, D., & von Larebeke, N. (2004). "Hormesis"—An inappropriate extrapolation from the specific to the universal. *International Journal of Occupational and Environmental Health 10*(3), 335–339.

Azarova, A., Irdam, D., Gugushvili, A. et al. (2017). The effect of rapid privatisation on mortality in mono-industrial towns in post-soviet Russia: A retrospective cohort study. *Lancet Public Health 2*(5), e231-e238.

Baldwin, J., & Grantham, V. (2015). Radiation hormesis: Historical and current perspectives. *Journal of Nuclear Medicine Technology 43*(4), 242–246.

Ball, H. (1986). Downwind from the bomb. *The New York Times Magazine* Feb. 9, 33.

Bard, D., Verger, P., & Hubert, P. (1997). Chernobyl, 10 years after: Health consequences. *Epidemiologic Reviews 19*(2), 187–204.

Baverstock, K., & Williams, D. (2006). The Chernobyl accident 20 years on: An assessment of the health consequences and the international response. *Environmental Health Perspectives 114*, 1312–1317.

https://doi.org/10.1515/9783110761788-021

Berkman, L. F., Kawachi, I., & Glymour, M. M. (Eds.) (2014). *Social epidemiology* (2nd ed.). Oxford; New York: Oxford University Press.

Beyea, J. (2017). Lessons to be learned from a contentious challenge to mainstream radiobiological science (the linear no-threshold theory of genetic mutations). *Environmental Research* 154, 362–379.

Bhattacharya, J., Gathmann, C., & Miller, G. (2013). The Gorbachev anti-alcohol campaign and Russia's mortality crisis. *American Economic Journal Applied Economics 5*(2), 232–260.

Black, S. E., Bütikofer, A., Devereux, P. J., & Salvanes, K. G. (2019). This is only a test? Long-run and intergenerational impacts of prenatal exposure to radioactive fallout. *Review of Economics and Statistics 101*(3), 531–546.

Blitz, M. (2016). When Kodak accidentally discovered A-bomb testing—Two thousand miles away from the U.S. A-bomb tests in 1945, something weird was happening to Kodak's film. *Popular Mechanics* (June 20).

Bochud, F. & Jung T. (2012), Comment on "The human sex odds at birth after the atmospheric atomic bomb tests, after Chernobyl, and in the vicinity of nuclear facilities". *Environmental Science and Pollution Research* 19:2456–2459.

Bonita, R., Beaglehole, R., & Kjelstroem, T. (2008). *Basic epidemiology* (2nd, corrected print out ed.). Geneva: World Health Organization.

Booth, C. (2020). Astonishing drinking sessions and epic hangovers in the world's booziest nation. *The Telegraph*, January 28.

Brainerd, E., & Cutler, D. M. (2005). Autopsy on an empire: Understanding mortality in Russia and the former Soviet Union. *Journal of Economic Perspectives 19*(1), 107–130.

Brenner, A. V., Tronko, M. D., Hatch, M. et al. (2012). I-131 dose response for incident thyroid cancers in Ukraine related to the Chornobyl accident. *Environmental Health Perspectives* 119(8), A332.

Brenner, D. J., Doll, R., Goodhead, D. T. et al. (2003). Cancer risks attributable to low doses of ionizing radiation: Assessing what we really know. *Proceedings of the National Academy of Sciences of the USA 100*(24), 13761.

Brodie, J. F. (2015). Radiation secrecy and censorship after Hiroshima and Nagasaki. *Journal of Social History 48*(4), 842–864.

Brown, K. (2019). *Manual for survival – A Chernobyl guide to the future.* New York: Norton.

Brown, K. (2013). *Plutopia: Nuclear families, atomic cities, and the great Soviet and American plutonium disasters.* Oxford: Oxford University Press.

Calabrese, E. J. (2005). Historical blunders: How toxicology got the dose-response relationship half right. *Cellular and Molecular Biology 51*(7), 643–654.

Calabrese, E. J. (2008). Astrocytes: Adaptive responses to low doses of neurotoxins. *Critical Reviews in Toxicology 38*(5), 463–471.

Calabrese, E. J. & Baldwin, L. A. (1999). The marginalization of hormesis. *Toxicological Pathology* 27(2), 187–194.

Calabrese, E. J., & Baldwin, L. A. (2001). The frequency of U-shaped dose responses in the toxicological literature. *Toxicological Sciences 62*(2), 330–338.

Calabrese, E. J., & Baldwin, L. A. (2001). Hormesis: A generalizable and unifying hypothesis. *Critical Reviews in Toxicology 31*(4–5), 353–424.

Calabrese, E. J., & Baldwin, L. A. (2002). Defining hormesis. *Human & Experimental Toxicology 21*(2), 91–97. doi:10.1191/0960327102ht217oa

Calabrese, E. J., & Baldwin, L. A. (2003). Toxicology rethinks its central belief. *Nature* *421*(6924), 691–692.

Cardis, E., Howe, R., Bebeshko, V., & Bogdanova, T. et al. (2006). Cancer consequences of the Chernobyl accident: 20 years on. *Journal of Radiological Protection 26*(2), 127–140.

Cardis, E., Krewski, D., Boniol, M., Drozdovitch, V. et al. (2006). Estimates of the cancer burden in Europe from radioactive fallout from the Chernobyl accident. *International Journal of Cancer, 119*(6), 1224–1235.

Case, A., & Deaton, D. (2015). Rising morbidity and mortality in midlife among white non-Hispanic Americans in the 21st century. *Proceedings of the National Academy of Sciences of the USA, 112*(49), 15078–15083.

Chernobyl Forum (2006). *Chernobyl's legacy: Health, environmental and socio-economic impacts, and recommendations to the governments of Belarus, the Russian federation and Ukraine.* Vienna: IAEA.

Clifford, C. (2022). Why the U.S. government plans to spend billions to keep money-losing nuclear plants open. *CNBC,* Feb 17. Retrieved March 2022 from www.cnbc.com/2022/02/17/the-us-is-spending-billions-to-keep-money-losing-nuclear-plants-open.html.

Cockerham, W. C. (Ed.) (1999). *Health and social change in Russia and Eastern Europe.* New York: Routledge.

Comar, C. L. (1963). *Fallout from nuclear tests.* Oak Ridge, TN: US Atomic Energy Commission.

Comprehensive Nuclear-Test-Ban Treaty Organization. 27 january 1951: The first of 904 nuclear tests conducted at the nevada nuclear test site. Retrieved March 2022 from www.ctbto.org/specials/who-we-are/

Cornia, G. A., & Paniccià, R. (Eds.) (2000). *The mortality crisis in transitional economies.* New York: Oxford University Press.

Cox, R., Muirhead, C. R., Stather, J. W., Edwards, A. A., & Little, M. P. (1995). *Risk of radiation-induced cancer at low doses and low dose ratesfor radiation protection purposes.* Chilton, Didcot, Oxfordshire: National Radiological Protection Board, UK.

Danzer, A. M., & Danzer, N. (2016). The long-run consequences of Chernobyl: Evidence on subjective well-being, mental health and welfare. *Journal of Public Economics 135*, 47–60.

Davis, S., Day, R., Kopecky, K., Mahoney, et al. International Consortium For Research On The Health Effects Of Radiation. Writing Committee and Study Team (2005). Childhood leukaemia in Belarus, Russia, and Ukraine following the Chernobyl power station accident: Results from an international collaborative population-based case–control study. *International Journal of Epidemiology 35*(2), 386–396. doi:10.1093/ije/dyi220

De Geer, L., Persson, C., & Rodhe, H. (2018). A nuclear jet at Chernobyl around 21:23:45 UTC on April 25, 1986. *Nuclear Technology 201*(1), 11–22.

de Vries, H., & Waterbolk, H. T. (1958). Groningen radiocarbon dates III. *Science 128*(3338), 1550–1556.

Dei, A. (2017), Hormesis and homeopathy—Toward a new self-consciousness. *Dose-Response* 15(4), 1–4.

Delongchamp, R. R., Mabuchi, K., Yoshimoto, Y., & Preston, D. L. (1997). Cancer mortality among atomic bomb survivors exposed in utero or as young children, October 1950-May 1992. *Radiation Research 147*(3), 385–395.

Dikov, I. (2018). How Bulgaria's communist regime hid the 1986 Chernobyl nuclear disaster from the public protecting only itself. paxglocalica.com/2018/04/26/how-bulgariascommunist-regime-hid-the-1986-chernobyl-nuclear-disaster-from-the-public-protecting-only-itself-written-for-archaeologyinbulgaria-com. Accessed February 2022.

Doll, R., & Hill, A. B. (1950). Smoking and carcinoma of the lung. *British Medical Journal* 2(4682), 739–748.

Dunning, G. M. (1955). Protecting the public during weapons testing at the Nevada test site. *JAMA 158*(11), 900–904.

Elliott, K. C. (2000). A case for caution: An evaluation of Calabrese and Baldwin's studies of chemical hormesis. *Risk 11*(2), 176–196.

Fabricant, J. I. (1981). The BEIR-III Report: Origin of the controversy. *American Journal of Roentgenology* 136, 209-214.Fabrikant, J. I. (1987). The Chernobyl disaster: An international perspective. *Industrial Crisis Quarterly, 1*(4), 2–12.

Fabrikant, J. I. (1991). The carcinogenic risks of low-LET and high-LET ionizing radiations. *Journal of Radiation Research 32*(2), 143–164.

Faden, R. (1996). The advisory committee on human radiation experiments: Reflections on a presidential commission. *The Hastings Center Report 26*(5), 5–10.

Fairlie, I., & Sumner, D. (2006). *The other report on Chernobyl (TORCH) – An independent scientific evaluation of the health-related effects of the Chernobyl nuclear disaster with critical analyses of recent IAEA/WHO reports*. Greens/EFA in the European Parliament. Retrieved February 2022 from cricket.biol.sc.edu/chernobyl/papers/TORCH.pdf

FDA. Fluoroscopy. Retrieved January 2022 from www.fda.gov/radiation-emitting-products/medical-x-ray-imaging/fluoroscopy

Feynman, R. P. (1998). *The meaning of it all – Toughts of a citizen scientist*. Reading, Mass.: Addison-Wesley.

Foner, E. (2006). *Give me liberty! An American history*. New York: W.W. Norton.

Fradkin, P. L. (1989). *Fallout: An American nuclear tragedy*. Tucson: University of Arizona Press.

Galea, S. (Ed.). (2007). *Macrosocial determinants of population health*. New York: Springer.

Gofman, J. W. (1990). Chapter 37 – Assessing Chernobyl's cancer consequences: Application of four 'Laws' of radiation carcinogenesis. Paper presented at the symposium on low-level radiation, national meeting of the American Chemical Society, September 9, 1986. In E. O'Connor (Ed.), *Radiation-induced cancer from low-dose exposure: An independent analysis*. San Francisco: Committee for Nuclear Responsibility.

Gofman, J. W. (1996). *Preventing breast cancer: The story of a major, proven, preventable cause of this disease*. San Francisco: Committee for Nuclear Responsibility.

Goldman, M., Catlin, R. J., & Anspaugh, L. (1987). *Health and environmental consequences of the Chernobyl nuclear power plant accident* (DOE/ER-0332 NTIS). Springfield. VA: US Department of Energy.

Grech, V. (2014). The Chernobyl accident, the male to female ratio at birth and birth rates. *Acta Medica 57*(2):62–67.

Greene, G. (2011). Richard Doll and Alice Stewart: Reputation and the shaping of scientific "truth". *Perspectives in Biology and Medicine 54*(4), 504–31.

Greene, G. (2017). *The woman who knew too much: Alice Stewart and the secrets of radiation* (2nd ed.). Ann Arbor: University of Michigan Press.

Grigoriev, P., & Andreev, E. M. (2015). The huge reduction in adult male mortality in Belarus and Russia: Is it attributable to anti-alcohol measures? *PLoS One 10*(9), e0138021.

Hatch, M. C., Beyea, J., Nieves, J. W., & Susser, M. (1990). Cancer near the Three Mile Island nudear plant: Radiation emissions. *American Journal of Epidemiology* 132(3), 392–412.

Hatch, M., Susser, M., & Beyea, J. (1997). Comments on "A reevaluation of cancer incidence near the Three Mile Island nuclear plant". *Environmental Health Perspectives 105*(1), 12.

Hatch, M. C., Wallenstein, S., Beyea, J., Nieves, J. W., & Susser, M. (1991). Cancer rates after the Three Mile Island nuclear accident and proximity of residence to the plant. *American Journal of Public Health 81*(6), 719–724.

Hatch, M., Ostroumova, E., Brenner, A., Federenko, Z. et al. (2015). Non-thyroid cancer in northern Ukraine in the post-Chernobyl period: Short report. *Cancer Epidemiology 39*(3), 279–283.

Hatch, M., & Cardis, E. (2017). Somatic health effects of Chernobyl: 30 years on. *European Journal of Epidemiology 32*(12), 1047–1054.

Haynes, M., & Husan, R. (2003). *A century of state murder? Death and policy in twentieth-century Russia*. London: Pluto Press.

Healio Hematology-Oncology. The shoe fitting fluoroscope, a little-known application of the X ray. Accessed April 2021 at www.healio.com/news/hematology-oncology/20120325/the-shoe-fitting-fluoroscope-a-little-known-application-of-the-x-ray.

Hoffmann, W. (2002). Has fallout from the Chernobyl accident caused childhood leukaemia in Europe? A commentary on the epidemiologic evidence. *European Journal of Public Health 12*(1), 72–76.

Honicker, C. T. (1987), *Premeditated deceit: The Atomic Energy Commission against Joseph August Sauter*. Dissertation for MA in Sociology, University of Tennessee, Knoxville. Accessed February 2022 at trace.tennessee.edu/utk_gradthes/4939/.

Hunnicutt, T., & Scheyderand, E.U.S. ban on Russian energy imports does not include uranium. *Reuters,* March 8, 2022. Retrieved April 2022 from www.reuters.com/business/energy/us-ban-russian-energy-imports-doesnt-include-uranium-source-2022-03-08/

IAEA (1991). *The international Chernobyl project: Assessment of radiological consequences and evaluation of protective measures – Report by an international advisory committee.* Vienna: International Atomic Energy Agency.

IAEA (1996). *After Chernobyl: What do we really know?* Vienna: International Atomic Energy Agency.

IAEA (2006). *Environmental consequences of the Chernobyl accident and their remediation: Twenty years of experience – Report of the Chernobyl Forum expert group "Environment"*. Vienna: International Atomic Energy Agency.

Ingram, M., Mason, W. B., Whipple, G. H., & Howland, J. W. (1952). *Biological effects of ionizing radiation – Sponsored by the US atomic energy commission [Declassified 3/15/13]*. Rochester, NY: University of Rochester. Retrieved December 2021 from https://www.osti.gov/servlets/purl/4389333

Ivanov, V. K. (2007). Late cancer and noncancer risks among Chernobyl emergency workers of Russia. *Health Physics 93*(5), 470–479.

Izrael, Y. A., De Cort, M., Jones, A. R., Nazarov, I. M. et al. (1996). The atlas of caesium-137 contamination of Europe after the Chernobyl accident. In A. Karaoglou, G. Desmet, G. N. Kelly & H. G. Menze (Eds.), *The radiological consequences of the Chernobyl accident – Proceedings of the first international conference, Minsk, Belarus, March 18–22, 1996* (pp. 1–10). Brussels: European Union.

Jacobson, M. Z. (2021a). *100 % clean, renewable energy and storage for everything*. New York: Cambridge University Press.

Jacobson, M. Z. (2021b). The 7 reasons why nuclear energy is not the answer to solve climate change. Retrieved April 2022 from eu.boell.org/en/2021/04/26/7-reasons-why-nuclear-energy-not-answer-solve-climate-change

Jargin, S. (2011). Thyroid cancer after Chernobyl: Obfuscated truth. *Dose-Response 9*, 471–476.

Jargin, S. V. (2014). Letter to the editor: On the radiation-leukemia dose-response relationship among recovery workers after the Chernobyl accident. *Dose-Response* 12(1), 162–165.

Jaworowski, Z. (2010). Observations on the Chernobyl disaster and LNT. *Dose-Response 8*(2), 148–171.

Joyce, C. WBUR news: Challenges loom large, 25 years after Chernobyl (April 26, 2011). Retrieved February 2021 from www.wbur.org/npr/135705270/challenges-loom-large-25-years-after-chernobyl

Kashcheev, V. V., Chekin, S. Y., Maksioutov, M. A., et al. (2015). Incidence and mortality of solid cancer among emergency workers of the chernobyl accident: Assessment of radiation risks for the follow-up period of 1992–2009. *Radiation and Environmental Biophysics 54*(1), 13–23.

Kesminiene, A., Evrard, A., Ivanov, V. K., Malakhova, I. V. et al. (2012). Risk of thyroid cancer among Chernobyl liquidators. *Radiation Research 178*(5), 425–436.

Kirsch, S. (2004). Harold Knapp and the geography of normal controversy: Radioiodine in the historical environment. *Osiris 19*, 167–181.

Kitchin, K. T., & Drane, J. W. (2005). A critique of the use of hormesis in risk assessment. *Human & Experimental Toxicology 24*(5), 249–253.

Knapp, H. (1964), Iodine-131 in fresh milk and human thyroids following a single deposition of nuclear test fall-out, *Nature* 202(4932), 534–537.

Knoll, G. F. (2010). *Radiation detection and measurement* (4th ed.). Hoboken, N.J.: John Wiley.

Kulakov, V. I., Sokur, T. N., Volobuev et al. (1993). Female reproductive function in areas affected by radiation after the Chernobyl power station accident. *Environmental Health Perspectives 101*, 117–123.

Kunitz, S. (1994). The value of particularism in the study of the cultural, social and behavioral determinants of mortality. In L. C. Chen, A. Kleinman & N. C. Ware (Eds.), *Health and social change in international perspective* (pp. 225–250). Boston: Harvard School of Public Health.

Kunitz, S. J. (2006). *The health of populations – General theories and particular realities*. New York: Oxford University Press.

Lehmann, H., & Wadsworth, J. (2011). The impact of Chernobyl on health and labour market performance. *Journal of Health Economics 30*(5), 843–857.

Lifton, R. J., & Mitchell, G. (1995). *Hiroshima in America: Fifty years of denial*. New York: Putnam.

Lim, H., Devesa, S. S., Sosa, J. A., Check, D., & Kitahara, C. M. (2017). Trends in thyroid cancer incidence and mortality in the United States, 1974–2013. *JAMA 317*(13), 1338–1348.

Little, M. P., Azizova, T. V., Bazyka, D. et al. (2012). Systematic review and meta-analysis of circulatory disease from exposure to low-level ionizing radiation and estimates of potential population mortality risks. *Environmental Health Perspectives 120*(11), 1503–1511.

Liubarets, T. F., Shibata, Y., Saenko, V. A., et al. (2019). Childhood leukemia in Ukraine after the Chornobyl accident. *Radiation and Environmental Biophysics 58*(4), 553–562.

Macalister, T., & Carter, H. (2009). Britain's farmers still restricted by Chernobyl nuclear fallout – Environmentalists say controls on 369 farms highlight danger of plans to build nuclear plants around UK. *The Guardian*, May 13.

Mackenbach, J. P. (2013). Political conditions and life expectancy in Europe, 1900–2008 *Social Science & Medicine* 82, 134–146.

Mahaffey, J. A. (2014). *Atomic accidents: A history of nuclear meltdowns and disasters: From the Ozark mountains to Fukushima*. New York: Pegasus Books.

Marino, F., & Nunziata, L. (2018). Long-term consequences of the Chernobyl radioactive fallout: An exploration of the aggregate data. *Milbank Quarterly 96*(4), 814–857.

Marples, D. R. (1996). The decade of despair. *Bulletin of the Atomic Scientists 52*(3), 20–31.

Mastauskas, A., Nedvecktaite, T., & Filistovic, V. (1997). *Consequences of the Chernobyl accident in lithuania*. International Atomic Energy Agency (IAEA): Retrieved December 2021 from http://inis.iaea.org/search/search.aspx?orig_q=RN:29013363

Mattson, M. P. (2008). Hormesis defined. *Ageing Research Review 7*(1), 1–7.

Meyers, K. (2019). In the shadow of the mushroom cloud: Nuclear testing, radioactive fallout, and damage to U.S. agriculture, 1945 to 1970. *Journal of Economic History 79*(1), 244–274.

Meyers, K. (2022). Some unintended fallout from defense policy: Measuring the effect of atmospheric nuclear testing on American mortality patterns [Working Paper, University of Southern Denmark, February 7]. Earlier draft available at squarespace.com/static/59262540b3db2b0d0d6d7d2b/t/5c81809a419202f922f0cfa4/1551990940274/FalloutMortDraft_3–5–2019.pdf

Michaelis, J., Haaf, H. G., Zöllner, J., Kaatsch, P., Krummenauer, F., & Berthold, F. (1996). Case control study of neuroblastoma in West Germany after the Chernobyl accident. *Klinische Pädiatrie 208*(4), 172–178.

Moysich, K. B., Menezes, R. J., & Michalek, A. M. (2002). Chernobyl-related ionising radiation exposure and cancer risk: An epidemiological review. *Lancet Oncology 3*(5), 269–279.

Mushak, P. (2007). Hormesis and its place in nonmonotonic dose-response relationships: Some scientific reality checks. *Environmental Health Perspectives* 15(4), 500–506.

NAS-NRC, National Academy of Sciences, National Research Council (1960). *The biological effects of atomic radiation – Summary report*. Washington DC: NAS/NSR.

National Research Council (1990). *Health effects of exposure to low levels of ionizing radiation: BEIR V*. Washington, DC: National Academies Press.

National Research Council (2006). *Health risks from exposure to low levels of ionizing radiation: BEIR VII phase 2*. Washington, DC: The National Academies Press.

National Research Council. (n.d.). BEIR VII: Health risks from exposure to low levels of ionizing radiation – report in brief. Retrieved November 2021 from dels.nas.edu/resources/static-assets/materials-based-on-reports/reports-in-brief/beir_vii_final.pdf

Nesterenko, A. B., Nesterenko, V. B., & Yablokov, A. V. (2009). Consequences of the Chernobyl catastrophe for public health. *Annals of the New York Academy of Sciences 1181*, 31–220.

Nesterenko, V. B., & Yablokov, A. V. (2009). Chernobyl contamination: An overview. *Annals of the New York Academy of Sciences 1181*, 4–30.

Nussbaum, R. H., & Kohnlein, W. (1994). Inconsistencies and open questions regarding low-dose health effects of ionizing radiation. *Environmental Health Perspectives 102*(8), 656–667.

Ostroumova, E., Hatch, M., Brenner, A., et al. (2016). Non-thyroid cancer incidence in Belarusian residents exposed to Chernobyl fallout in childhood and adolescence: Standardized incidence ratio analysis, 1997–2011. *Environmental Research 147*, 44–49.

Parker, S. P. (1984). *McGraw-hill dictionary of physics*. New York: McGraw-Hill.

Parsons, M. A. (2014). *Dying unneeded: The cultural context of the Russian mortality crisis*. Nashvile: Vanderbilt University Press.

Pauling, L. (1983). *No more war! [1st ed. 1958]*. New York: Dodd, Mead.

Peplow, M. (2006). Counting the dead: Twenty years after the worst nuclear accident in history, arguments over the death toll of Chernobyl are as politically charged as ever. *Nature 440*(7087), 982–983.

Petridou, E., Trichopoulos, D., Dessypris, N., et al. (1997). Infant leukaemia after in utero exposure to radiation from chernobyl. *Nature 387*(6630), 246.

Petridou, E., Proukakis, C., Tong, et al. D. (1994). Trends and geographical distribution of childhood leukemia in Greece in relation to the Chernobyl accident. *Scandinavian Journal of Social Medicine 22*(2), 127–131.

Pitkevitch, V. A., Ivanov, V. K., Tsyb, A. F. et al. (1997). Exposure levels for persons involved in recovery operations after the Chernobyl accident: Statistical analysis based on the data of the Russian National Medical and Dosimetric Registry. *Radiation and Environmental Biophysics, 36*(3), 149–160.

Plokhy, S. (2019). The Chernobyl cover-up: How officials botched evacuating an irradiated city. Retrieved October 2021 from www.history.com/news/chernobyl-disaster-coverup.

Poch, R. (2017). La disolución de la URSS. *La Vanguardia* (Barcelona), December 6.

Pohl-Rüling, J., Haas, O. A., Obe, G. et al. (1990). The Chernobyl fallout in Salzburg, Austria, and its effect on blood chromosomes. *Acta Biologica Hungarica 41*(1–3), 215–222.

Polednak, A. D. (1978). Bone cancer among female radium dial workers – Latency periods and incidence rates by time after exposure. *Journal of the National Cancer Institute 60*(1), 77–82.

Pukkala, E., Kesminiene, A., Poliakov et al. (2006). Breast cancer in Belarus and Ukraine after the Chernobyl accident. *International Journal of Cancer 119*(3), 651–658.

Radiopaedia. Thomas Edison. Accessed January 2022 at radiopaedia.org/articles/thomas-edison/changesets/307845/edits?lang=us.

Revkin, A. C. (2013). Dot earth: 'To those influencing environmental policy but opposed to nuclear power'. November 3. Retrieved March 2022 from https://dotearth.blogs.nytimes.com/2013/11/03/to-those-influencing-environmental-policy-but-opposed-to-nuclear-power/

Rice, J. (2015). Downwind of the atomic state: US continental atmospheric testing, radioactive fallout, and organizational deviance, 1951–1962. *Social Science History 39*(4), 647–676.

Ricarte-Filho J. C., Li, S., Garcia-Rendueles, M. E. R. et al. (2013). Identification of kinase fusion oncogenes in post-Chernobyl radiation-induced thyroid cancers. *Journal of Clinical Investigation 123*(11), 4935–4944.

Richmond, C. (2002). Alice Mary Stewart. *BMJ 325*(7355), 106–106.

Ringholz, R. C. (2002). *Uranium frenzy: Saga of the nuclear west.* Logan, Utah: Utah State University Press.

Riphahn, R. T., & Zimmermann, K. F. (2000). The mortality crisis in East Germany. In G. A. Cornia, & R. Paniccià (Eds.), *The mortality crisis in transitional economies* (pp. 227–252). New York: Oxford University Press.

Rodgers, B. E., & Holmes, K. M. (2008). Radio-adaptive response to environmental exposures at Chernobyl. *Dose-Response 6*(2), 209–221.

Rosefield, S. (2001). Premature deaths: Russia's radical economic transition in Soviet perspective. *Europe-Asia Studies 53*(8), 1159–1176.

Roszkowska, H., & Goryński, P. (2004). [Thyroid cancer in Poland in 1980–2000] [in Polish]. *Przegląd Epidemiologiczny 58*(2), 369–76.

Russell, W. L., Russell, L. B., & Kelly, E. M. (1958). Radiation dose rate and mutation frequency. *Science 128*(3338), 1546–1550.

Sachs, J. D. (2009). Shock therapy' had no adverse effect on life expectancy in Eastern Europe. *Financial Times* Jan 19.

Sacks, B., Meyerson, G., & Siegel, J. A. (2016). Epidemiology without biology: False paradigms, unfounded assumptions, and specious statistics in radiation science (with commentaries by Inge Schmitz-Feuerhake and Christopher Busby and a reply by the authors). *Biological Theory 11*, 69–101.

Sagan, L. A. (1987). What is hormesis and why haven't we heard about it before? *Health Physics 52*(5), 521–525.

Samet, J. M., de González, A. B., Dauer, L. T., Hatch, M., Kosti, O., Mettler, J.,Fred A., & Satyamitra, M. M. (2018). Gilbert W. Beebe symposium on 30 years after the Chernobyl accident: Current and future studies on radiation health effects. *Radiation Research 189*(1), 5–18.

Satter, D. (2017). *The less you know, the better you sleep: Russia's road to terror and dictatorship under Yeltsin and Putin.* New Haven: Yale University Press.

Schmemann, S. (1986). Soviet announces nuclear accident at electric plant. *New York Times*, April 29, A1–A6.

Scherb, H. & Voigt, K. (2011). The human sex odds at birth after the atmospheric atomic bomb tests, after Chernobyl, and in the vicinity of nuclear facilities. *Environmental Science and Pollution Research* 18:697–707

Scherb, H. & Voigt, K. (2012). Response to F. Bochud and T. Jung. *Environmental Science & Pollution Research* 19:4234–4241.

Shrader-Frechette, K. (2008). Ideological toxicology: Invalid logic, science, ethics about low-dose pollution. *Human & Experimental Toxicology 27*(8), 647–657.

Shrader-Frechette, K. (2012). Research integrity and conflicts of interest: The case of unethical research-misconduct charges filed by Edward Calabrese. *Accountability in Research 19*(4), 220–242.

Siegel, J. A., Sacks, B., & Greenspan, B. S. (2018). There is no evidence to support the Linear No-Threshold model of radiation carcinogenesis. *Journal of Nuclear Medicine 59*(12), 1918.

Simon, S. L., Bouville, A., & Land, C. E. (2006). Fallout from nuclear weapons tests and cancer risks: Exposures 50 years ago still have health implications today that will continue into the future. *American Scientist 94*(1), 48–57.

Simons, M. (1993). Soviet atom test used thousands as guinea pigs, archives show. *New York Times*, Nov. 7, pp. 1 & 20. Retrieved January 2022 from www.nytimes.com/1993/11/07/world/soviet-atom-test-used-thousands-as-guinea-pigs-archives-show.html

Sofia Globe staff (2020). Bulgaria, April 1986: The Chernobyl cover-up. *The Sofia Globe* April 26. Accessed February 2022 sofiaglobe.com/2020/04/26/bulgaria-april-1986-the-chernobyl-cover-up/.

Sterling, P., & Platt, M. L. (2022). Why deaths of despair are increasing in the US and not other industrial Nations—Insights from neuroscience and anthropology. *JAMA Psychiatry* 79(4), 368–374.

Stevens, W., Thomas, D. C., Lyon, J. L. et al. (1990). Leukemia in Utah and radioactive fallout from the Nevada test site: A case-control study. *Journal of the American Medical Association* 264(94), 585–591.

Stillman, S. (2006). Health and nutrition in eastern europe and the former soviet union during the decade of transition: A review of the literature. *Economics & Human Biology* 4(1), 104–146.

Stsjazhko, V. A., Tsyb, A. F., Tronko, N. D., Souchkevitch, G., & Baverstock, K. F. (1995). Childhood thyroid cancer since accident at Chernobyl [letter]. *BMJ 310*(6982), 801.

Stuckler, D., & Basu, S. (2013). How austerity kills. *New York Times*, May 13, A19.

Stuckler, D., King, L., & McKee, M. (2009). Mass privatization and the post-communist mortality crisis. *Lancet, 373*, 399–407.

Suddath, C. (2010). A brief history of Russians and vodka. *Time* January 5. Retrieved January 2022 from web.archive.org/web/20100525170240/http://www.time.com/time/world/article/0%2C8599%2C1951620%2C00.html

Svendsen, E. R., Kolpakov, I. E., Stepanova, Y. I. et al. (2010). ^{137}Cesium exposure and spirometry measures in Ukrainian children affected by the Chernobyl nuclear incident. *Environmental Health Perspectives* 118(5), 720–725.

Talbott, E. O., Youk, A. O., McHugh, K. P., et al (2000a). Mortality among the residents of the Three Mile Island accident area: 1979–1992. *Environmental Health Perspectives* 108(6), 545–552.

Talbott, E. O., Youk, A. O., McHugh, K. P., et al (2000b). Re: "Collision of evidence and assumptions: TMI déjà view" [letter]. *Environmental Health Perspectives* 108(12), A547-A549.

Tapia Granados, J. A. (2013). Repression, famines, and wars: Major impacts of politics on population health. *Social Science & Medicine* 86, 103–106.

Tomka, B. (2013). *A social history of twentieth-century Europe*. New York: Routledge.

Tomonaga, M. (1962). Leukaemia in Nagasaki atomic bomb survivors from 1945 through 1959. *Bulletin of the World Health Organization 26*(5), 619–631.

Tondel, M., Lindgren, P., Hjalmarsson, P., Hardell, L., & Persson, B. (2006). Increased incidence of malignancies in Sweden after the Chernobyl accident – A promoting effect? *American Journal of Industrial Medicine* 49(3), 159–68.

Tondel, M., Hjalmarsson, P., Hardell, L., Carlsson, G., & Axelson, O. (2004). Increase of regional total cancer incidence in north Sweden due to the Chernobyl accident? *Journal of Epidemiology & Community Health* 58, 1011.

Truman, H. S. President Harry Truman announces the bombing of Hiroshima. Retrieved November 2021 from www.youtube.com/watch?v=FN_UJJ9ObDs

Udall, S. (1994). *The myths of August: A personal exploration of our tragic Cold War affair with the atom.* New York: Pantheon/Random House.

United States Congress, Joint Committee on Atomic Energy, Special Subcommittee on Radiation. (1957). *Summary-analysis of hearings may 27–29, and june 3–7, 1957, The nature of radioactive fallout and its effects on man.* Washington: Government Printing Office. Retrieved November 2021 from https://www.heinonline.org/HOL/Page?handle=hein.cbhear/cbhearings10874&id=1&size=2&collection=congrec&index=cbhear;

United States Congress, Joint Committee on Atomic Energy, Special Subcommittee on Radiation. (1958). *The nature of radioactive fallout and its effects on man.* Washington: Government Printing Office. Retrieved November 2021 from https://www.heinonline.org/HOL/Page?handle=hein.cbhear/cbhearings10874&id=1&size=2&collection=congrec&index=cbhear

University of California, Berkeley, Max Planck Institute for Demographic Research. *Human mortality database,* www.mortality.org

UNSCEAR (1988). *Sources, effects and risks of ionizing radiation: United Nations Scientific Committee on the Effects of Atomic Radiation 1988 report to the General Assembly, with annexes.* New York: United Nations Scientific Committee on the Effects of Atomic Radiation.

UNSCEAR. (1993). *Sources and effects of ionizing radiation: United Nations Scientific Committee on the Effects of Atomic Radiation 1993 report to the General Assembly, with annexes.* New York: United Nations Scientific Committee on the Effects of Atomic Radiation.

UNSCEAR. (2000). *Sources and effects of ionizing radiation: UNSCEAR 2000 report to the general assembly.* New York: United Nations Scientific Committee on the Effects of Atomic Radiation.

UNSCEAR. (2008). The Chernobyl accident: UNSCEAR's assessments of the radiation effects. Retrieved January 2022 from www.unscear.org/unscear/en/chernobyl.html

US Congress, House Committee on Interstate and Foreign Commerce, Subcommittee on Oversight and Investigations. (1980). *Low-level radiation effects on health: Hearings before the Subcommittee on Oversight and Investigations of the Committee on Interstate and Foreign Commerce, House of Representatives, 96th Congress, 5th session, April 23, May 24, and August 1, 1979.* Washington, DC: US Government Printing Office.

Vapirev, E. I., Georgiev, G., Jordanov, T., & Hristova, A. V. (1996). Estimation of the total fallout of Sr-90 and Cs-137 over the territory of Bulgaria after the Chernobyl accident. *Bulgarian Journal of Physics 23*(3/4), 129–147.

Wedel, J.R. (2001). *Collision and collusion: The strange case of western aid to Eastern Europe.* New York: St. Martins Press.

WHO (2016). 1986–2016: Chernobyl at 30 – An update. Retrieved January 2022 from https://www.who.int/ionizing_radiation/chernobyl/Chernobyl-update.pdf

WHO Regional Office for Europe. European Health for All Database (HFA-DB), www.euro.who.int/hfadb

Wikipedia. Chernobyl disaster. Retrieved October 2021 from en.wikipedia.org/wiki/Chernobyl_disaster.

Wikipedia. Linear no threshold model. Accessed July 2021 at en.wikipedia.org/wiki/Linear_no-threshold_model.

Wikipedia. Pierre Curie. Accessed January 2022 at en.wikipedia.org/wiki/Pierre_Curie.

Wikipedia. Shoe-fitting fluoroscope. Accessed April 2021 at en.wikipedia.org/wiki/Shoe-fitting_fluoroscope.

Wikipedia. Yury Bandazhevsky. Accessed April 2021 at en.wikipedia.org/wiki/Yury_Bandazhevsky.

Williams, D., & Baverstock, K. (2006). Too soon for a final diagnosis: *Nature 440*, 993–994.

Williams, D. (2002). Cancer after nuclear fallout: Lessons from the Chernobyl accident. *Nature Reviews Cancer 2*(7), 543.

Wing, S., & Richardson, D. (2000). Collision of evidence and assumptions: TMI déjà view [letter]. *Environmental Health Perspectives 108*(12), A546-A547.

Wing, S., Richardson, D., Armstrong, D., & Crawford-Brown, D. (1997). A reevaluation of cancer incidence near the Three Mile Island nuclear plant: The collision of evidence and assumptions. *Environmental Health Perspectives 105*(1), 52–57.

Yablokov, A. V. & Nesterenko, V. B. (2009). Chernobyl contamination through time and space. *Annals of the New York Academy of Sciences* 1181, 4–30, 14.

Yemelyanau, M., Amialchuk, A., & Ali, M. M. (2012). Evidence from the Chernobyl nuclear accident: The effect on health, education, and labor market outcomes in Belarus. *Journal of Labor Research 33*(1), 1–20.

Zablotska, L. B., Bazyka, D., Lubin, J. H., et al. (2013). Radiation and the risk of chronic lymphocytic and other leukemias among Chornobyl cleanup workers. *Environmental Health Perspectives 121*(1), 59–65.

Index

https://doi.org/10.1515/9783110761788-022

www.ingramcontent.com/pod-product-compliance
Lightning Source LLC
Chambersburg PA
CBHW070906100426
42737CB00047B/2870